LIVING with HEMOCHROMATOSIS

Expert Answers to Your Questions about Iron Overload

GREGORY T. EVERSON, MD, FACP
and HEDY WEINBERG

A HEALTHY LIVING BOOK

New York

LIVING WITH HEMOCHROMATOSIS:
Expert Answers to Your Questions about Iron Overload

GREGORY T. EVERSON, MD, FACP
HEDY WEINBERG

A Healthy Living Book
Hatherleigh Press
5-22 46th Avenue
Long Island City, NY 11101
1-800-528-2550

DISCLAIMER
This book does not give legal or medical advice.
Always consult your doctor, lawyer, and other professionals.
The names of people who contributed anecdotal material have been changed.

Names of medications are typically followed by ™ or ® symbols, but these symbols are not stated in this book.

The ideas and suggestions contained in this book are not intended as a substitute for consulting with a physician. All matters regarding your health require medical supervision.

Library of Congress Cataloging-in-Publication Data
Everson, Gregory T., 1950–
      Living with hemochromatosis : answers to questions about iron overload /
Gregory Everson and Hedy Weinberg.
              p. cm.
      Includes bibliographical references.
      ISBN 1-57826-104-X (alk. paper)
      1. Hemochromatosis—Popular works. I. Weinberg, Hedy, 1939- II. Title.

RC632.H4E946 2003
616.3'9042—dc21
                                                          2003050871

All Hatherleigh Press titles are available for special promotions and premiums.
For more information, please contact the manager of our Special Sales department.

Cover design by Tai Blanche
Printed in Canada on acid-free paper
10 9 8 7 6 5 4 3 2 1

DEDICATION

To all the people and families who eloquently shared their stories about the struggles and triumphs of living with hereditary hemochromatosis

With special thanks to:

Sandra Thomas, President and Founder of the American Hemochromatosis Society, and the members of Families HHelping Families Circle, the AHS online support group;

Debby McVay and the members of the Hemochromatosis Support Group at Swedish Medical Center in Denver, Colorado;

Patients and staff at the University of Colorado Health Sciences Center, Section of Hepatology, Liver Disease and Transplantation

GREGORY T. EVERSON, MD, FACP
HEDY WEINBERG

CONTENTS

PREFACE IX

ACKNOWLEDGMENTS XI

FOREWORD XIII
By BRUCE R. BACON, M.D., Director,
Division of Gastroenterology and Hepatology
Saint Louis University Liver Center

1. WHAT IS HEMOCHROMATOSIS? 1
An Introduction

2. WHEN YOU HAVE HEMOCHROMATOSIS 13
Blood Tests, Liver Biopsy, and Other Diagnostic Tests

3. GENETIC (DNA) TESTS 30
What Do They Mean?

4. THE CARRIER 47
What About Me? What About My Family?

5. HOW HEMOCHROMATOSIS
DAMAGES YOUR BODY 65
*Effects of Iron Overload on the Liver, Heart, Pancreas,
Joints, and Endocrine System*

6. TAKING CARE OF YOURSELF NUTRITIONALLY 78
Guidelines for Healthy Nutrition in Hemochromatosis

7. TAKING CARE OF YOURSELF EMOTIONALLY 98
Coping with a Genetic Condition

8. FINANCIAL IMPACT OF HEMOCHROMATOSIS 122
Treatment Costs and Insurance Factors

9. TREATMENT FOR HEMOCHROMATOSIS 143
   Phlebotomy and Other Issues

10. LIVER CANCER (HEPATOMA) 156
   Are You at Risk?

11. LIVER TRANSPLANTS FOR
    HEMOCHROMATOSIS 171
   A Medical Miracle

12. RESEARCH TRENDS 194
   Hope for the Future

RESOURCES 202

SELECTED CITATIONS 206

INDEX 224

PREFACE

SOME MONTHS AFTER THE PUBLICATION OF THE third edition of our *Living with Hepatitis C* and the first edition of *Living with Hepatitis B*, Kevin Moran called to say that Hatherleigh Press would like to add a book on hemochromatosis (HH) to the series. At first, I declined because of an extremely busy schedule.

But Kevin persisted. He said he had a friend who was recently diagnosed with HH, and Kevin was astounded to learn that more than one million people in the U.S. have hereditary hemochromatosis. One in 10 people are carriers. In other words, 25 to 30 million Americans have gene mutations for HH.

Again, I hesitated. My schedule was still crowded, and several patient guides for HH were already on the market. In what way would our book be different? What could we add that would help our readers?

I finally decided that I could make a contribution and add to the existing literature in two areas:

(1) Because hemochromatosis primarily targets the liver, I offer a hepatologist's unique perspective on liver disease caused by HH.

(2) My goal is to present complex medical terms in language that patients can understand—a particular challenge when dealing with complicated genetic material. I hope that I have succeeded.

In these pages you will hear from patients and staff at the University Hospital and the University of Colorado Health Sciences Center who generously contributed their knowledge and experiences. In addition, people and families from all around the country shared their stories in order to help others cope with HH.

With the mapping of the human genome, our understanding of HH will continue to grow. Throughout the book I emphasize the need for thoughtful well-controlled clinical and basic research of hereditary hemochromatosis. The final chapter speculates on potential scientific and medical breakthroughs.

I hope that this book will help patients and doctors avoid the unfortunate pitfalls of delayed diagnosis. Hemochromatosis, when diagnosed early, is treatable, and patients who are identified before iron accumulates in their organs can expect to live a full and normal lifespan.

One last word: Although *Living with Hemochromatosis: Answers to Questions about Iron Overload* is a detailed reference guide, it does not replace the advice and care of your physician, nor does it give legal advice. Instead, it is designed solely to educate patients and their families about hereditary hemochromatosis and how it affects their lives. Consult appropriate specialists, and always work closely with your doctor when making medical decisions.

GREGORY T. EVERSON, M.D., F.A.C.P.

ACKNOWLEDGMENTS

WE APPRECIATE AND GRATEFULLY ACKNOWL-edge the hard-working, dedicated members of the Liver Team at the University of Colorado Health Sciences Center, who are always generous with help and support: James Trotter, M.D.; Marcelo Kugelmas, M.D.; Lisa Forman, M.D.; Paul Hayashi, M.D.; Greg Fitz, M.D.; Igal Kam, M.D., Chief of Division of Transplant Surgery; Michael Wachs, M.D.; Thomas Bak, M.D.; Susan Mandell, M.D.; Thomas Beresford, M.D.; Barbara Fey, R.N., M.S.N., Hepatology Nurse; Cathy Ray, R.N., B.S.N., M.A., Hepatology Nurse; Anne Shaver, R.N., B.S.N., Hepatology Nurse; Megan Dyer, Lori Carrillo, Administrative Assistants; Donna Cornelisse, C.M.A., Medical Technologist; Dawn Schmidt, Medical Assistant; Jennifer DeSanto, R.N., Research Coordinator; Brenda Martin, R.N., Research Coordinator; Carol McKinley, R.N., Research Coordinator; Sue Sellissen, P.R.A.; Shannon Lauriski; Christy Kennedy; Tracy Steinberg, R.N., M.S., C.C.T.C.; Tim Brackett, R.N.; Mary McClure, R.N.; Michael Talamantes, M.S.S.W., L.C.S.W.

Also from the University of Colorado Health Sciences Center, we give special thanks to Carol Walton, M.S., C.G.C., Director, Graduate Program in Genetic Counseling, Instructor, Department of Pediatrics, for her help with emotional issues arising from genetic conditions and for her expertise on the issues of genetic discrimination; Paul Seligman, M.D., Professor of Medicine, Division of Hematology and Oncology, for his expertise and special interest in hereditary hemochromatosis; Robert M. House, M.D., Associate Professor, Director, Residency Training, Department of Psychiatry; Hannis W. Thompson, M.D., Director of Transfusion Medicine, Associate Professor of Pathology; Fabi Imo, Coordinator, Transplant Financial Services; Patty Polski, M.B.A., Manager,

Registration and Financial Services ; Rev. Julie Swaney, University Hospital Chaplain.

Dr. Everson wishes to further acknowledge the support of the staff at University Hospital and the University of Colorado Health Sciences Center in the care and management of patients with hemochromatosis.

We thank Meredith Pate-Willig, M.S.W., L.C.S.W., for her invaluable help with the emotional challenges of chronic illness; Annette K. Taylor, M.S., Ph.D., President and Laboratory Director, and Karen Montgomery, M.S., of Kimball Genetics for their generous assistance with issues concerning genetic testing.

Special thanks to Sandra Thomas, President and Founder of the American Hemochromatosis Society, and the members of Families HHelping Families Circle, the AHS online support group; Debby McVay and the members of the Hemochromatosis Support Group at Swedish Medical Center in Denver, Colorado; and patients at the University of Colorado Health Sciences Center, Section of Hepatology, Liver Disease and Transplantation, for sharing their stories and insights about living with hemochromatosis.

FOREWORD

Physicians and scientists have known about hemochromatosis for almost 140 years. A French physician, Trousseau, is credited with the first description of the disease in 1865, and the famous German pathologist, von Recklinghausen, first used the term "hemochromatosis" in 1889, thinking it was a pigment disorder (chrom) of the blood (hemo). In 1935, Joseph Sheldon, a British gerontologist, wrote a monograph cataloging all 311 cases of hemochromatosis that had been reported up to that time. Despite having no modern molecular techniques available to him, he correctly concluded that hemochromatosis was an inherited disorder in which all of the pathological findings developed as a result of excess iron deposits in tissues.

In 1976, a French geneticist, Marcel Simon, demonstrated definitively that the gene for hemochromatosis was located on the short arm of chromosome 6 within the genetically rich HLA region of the genome. Despite this general localization, it was another twenty years before a team of molecular geneticists at a small biotech company, Mercator Genetics, identified the gene and the principle mutations that are responsible for hemochromatosis. Following this discovery, an explosion of new knowledge about iron absorption, iron transport, and regulation of iron homeostasis has come about. The use of mutation analysis (i.e., gene test) has improved diagnosis in individuals, replaced HLA testing in family studies, and is being considered for large-scale population studies.

With all of this new scientific information about hemochromatosis that has come forward over the last seven years, it is fitting that a book for patients has been written. Dr. Gregory Everson, a noted hepatologist at the University of Colorado, along with Hedy Weinberg, a medical writer, have created a masterpiece, *Living with Hemochromatosis: Expert Answers to Your Questions About Iron Overload*. Following on their earlier success with *Living with Hepatitis C: A Survivor's Guide* (now in its 3rd edition) and *Living with Hepatitis B*, Dr. Everson and Ms. Weinberg have created another excellent work for patients. All areas of hemochromatosis have been covered: from diagnostic testing, including genetic tests, to mechanisms of how iron overload is injurious to cells, tissues and organs; from nutritional recommendations and support for emotional issues to treatment, including transplant. The book concludes with new areas of research. Each chapter is populated with colorful anecdotes provided by patients that give realistic information for the reader.

As in the other books by these authors, the information provided is accurate and authoritative. More importantly, complicated scientific and medical concepts are beautifully explained in clear detail so that patients and non-medical personnel can easily understand them. This book meets its expectations and will find an important niche for patients and families who are afflicted by this common genetic disease—hemochromatosis. The authors are to be congratulated!

BRUCE R. BACON, M.D.
James F. King MD Endowed Chair in Gastroenterology
Professor of Internal Medicine
Director, Division of Gastroenterology and Hepatology
Saint Louis University Liver Center
Saint Louis University School of Medicine
Saint Louis, Missouri

1

WHAT IS HEMOCHROMATOSIS?

An Introduction

Gold is for the mistress—silver for the maid—
Copper for the craftsman cunning at his trade.
"Good!" said the Baron, sitting in his hall,
"But Iron—Cold Iron—is master of them all."
Cold Iron
RUDYARD KIPLING

I F YOU'VE JUST BEEN DIAGNOSED WITH HEMO-
chromatosis, you have a lot of questions: "What is hemochromatosis? How did I get it?"

Hereditary hemochromatosis (HH), also known as hereditary
human hemochromatosis (HHC), is a disorder caused by specific
genetic mutations that allow your body to retain too much iron. That's
why we also call hemochromatosis "Iron Overload." Actually, HH is
only one of several iron overload conditions, but it is the most common. Mutations that lead to hemochromatosis tend to occur in a single
gene, the HFE gene.

At this point, you may be saying, "Wait a minute. I thought iron was
good for me. TV commercials and ads boast that cereals and tonics are
fortified with iron. How can I have too much of a good thing?"

The answer is both simple and complicated. Iron is a nutrient that your cells must have in order to survive, but you only need about 1 to 2 milligrams per day. If you have the normal HFE gene, your body won't absorb more than the amount needed. When you have the mutation in the HFE gene (HH), your body absorbs excessive amounts of iron. Iron accumulates in your cells, and your body lacks the mechanisms to remove the excess iron. Over time, this iron buildup damages not only cells and tissues but also organs.

Hemochromatosis primarily targets the liver, but iron accumulation also can harm other organs, including the pancreas, heart, joints, and hormonal system. Obviously, the potential for injury to all these organs may make you feel apprehensive and concerned. Remember, this condition progresses very slowly. If detected at an early stage, organ damage and its complications can be avoided. The good news is that today we have tests that can diagnose you early—before organ damage occurs.

Treatment is safe and effective. Although your body absorbs excessive iron and retains it, you can get rid of the iron through blood loss by periodic blood removal (phlebotomy). If you are diagnosed early, phlebotomy may be all the treatment you need. However, if you have advanced hemochromatosis that has already affected body organs, you may have to treat the diseased organs in addition to regular phlebotomy treatments. For example, if your pancreas has been damaged, your doctor may prescribe insulin for diabetes.

As you can see, patients with hemochromatosis face varied problems. Some people will be detected, treated early, and therefore will avoid any symptoms, signs, or clinical problems. Others will be diagnosed late, after organ damage has occurred, and will face not only the need for phlebotomy but also the challenges of treatments to preserve organ function or reverse organ damage. The goals of this book are to guide you through the whole spectrum of HH—from early to delayed diagnosis—and to answer your questions about living with hemochromatosis.

Cases of hemochromatosis were recorded more than 120 years ago. But researchers didn't discover the HFE gene and its mutations that cause hemochromatosis until 1996. With today's genetic studies, we now know that HH is not a rare condition. In fact, according to the CDC, hemochromatosis is one of the most common genetic disorders in humans.

Current studies indicate that hereditary hemochromatosis originated in populations of Northern European ancestry. An extremely high incidence is found in Ireland and in other Celtic populations, such as Wales, Australia, and areas in the U.S. and Canada where Irish immigrants settled. The high prevalence in Iceland may also be linked to early Celtic inhabitants of this island. Some scientists suggest that the HH mutation aided survival in places where nutritional sources of iron were scarce.

> *In 1981 I was feeling tired. There was a history of diabetes in my family so I went to the doctor. At that time, they weren't routinely checking for iron, but for some reason the lab did run a test. Turned out I had a very high iron load.*
>
> *My ancestors are all from England except for one great grandmother from Switzerland. Some diseases are advantageous to society. My English ancestors didn't need as much meat because they absorbed a lot of iron from the meat they had. So while others died, my ancestors were hopping around. Mother Nature doesn't care how long you live, only that you live long enough to reproduce.*
>
> MIKE

One theory concerning the high frequency of HH in the Celtic population hypothesizes that people with HH gene mutations enjoyed a survival advantage over the unaffected population by preventing iron deficiency. Iron deficiency in women of childbearing age is associated with impaired work performance, intolerance to exercise, impaired energy metabolism, and adverse outcome of pregnancy.

Dr. Christian Datz and his colleagues from Salzburg, Austria, studied 468 healthy women between the ages of 18 to 40. Two had HH and 44 were carriers. Iron studies in the 44 carriers and unaffected women indicated that carriers had higher hemoglobin and iron levels. According to Dr. Datz, "We feel that the high frequency of mutations in the hemochromatosis gene may result from a selection advantage, conferring protection against iron deficiency in young women."

A Word of Caution: Information in this book does not substitute for the advice of your physician. If you have hemochromatosis, you should be under a doctor's care.

In this chapter we'll discuss some basic facts and statistics about hemochromatosis, its symptoms, history and discovery. Here are the topics we'll cover:

- ◆ *You Are Not Alone*
- ◆ *Signs and Symptoms*
- ◆ *The Discovery of Hemochromatosis*

+ *Understanding Hemochromatosis*
    WHAT IS IRON?
    WHAT IS A GENETIC MUTATION?
    WHO HAS HEMOCHROMATOSIS?
    WHO IS A CARRIER?
+ *Other Conditions of Iron Overload (Not Hemochromatosis)*
+ *Hemochromatosis: Early Detection Is the Key*

You Are Not Alone

I had no idea what hemochromatosis meant at the time I was diagnosed. It wasn't until I hooked up with an online support group that I learned 80 percent of what I know from a couple of members who do a lot of research. If you don't have a support system, you feel as if you're on a desert island, because so few people have heard of hemochromatosis.

CHRISTINE

It may help to know that you're not alone. According to the Centers for Disease Control and Prevention (CDC), as many as one million people living in the United States have evidence of hemochromatosis. These affected Americans carry two mutated HFE genes. Many more Americans are silent carriers. One in 10 people are carriers, meaning that they carry one mutated HFE gene. In other words, 25 to 30 million Americans have HFE gene mutations. We now know that some carriers also may have iron overload, although typically to a lesser degree and severity. It may surprise you to learn that the number of people in the United States with hereditary hemochromatosis is greater than the estimated number of people with HIV/AIDS.

As stated above, hereditary hemochromatosis is due to inheritance of two mutations of the HFE gene. The most common genetic mutation, C282Y, is the most common cause of hereditary hemochromatosis and affects between 1 in 200 to 1 in 250 people with Northern European ancestry. An extremely high incidence is found in Ireland and other Celtic populations where the prevalence of HH may be as much as 1 in 100. Analysis of prevalence of the mutations of the HFE gene indicates that the C282Y mutation may have originated in the Celtic areas of Northern Europe.

About ten to fifteen years ago, my doctor noted that my blood tests were high in iron. He mentioned hemochromatosis, but I had never heard of it. I started asking my relatives. A great-aunt on my mother's side had been diagnosed with HH. Every one of my older relatives died of heart disease—my grandmother at age 46. And she didn't smoke or have any other risk factors.

You don't hear about hemochromatosis very much, but I remembered reading that people of Celtic origin have a high frequency of HH. And my dad always likes to say that we're 150 percent Welsh!

KAREN

Numbers and statistics, however, don't begin to describe the impact of HH on people's lives. When you're diagnosed with hemochromatosis, you are concerned about yourself and about the people in your family who may have HH or who may be carriers. You have new issues to consider: dealing with phlebotomy treatments, telling family members about the genetic nature of HH, and coping with symptoms of hemochromatosis.

Signs and Symptoms

Hemochromatosis is a metallic time bomb. Deposits of iron silently build in the body over decades. That's why most symptoms associated with hemochromatosis appear more frequently in middle age (but can occur at younger ages). In addition, diagnosis is often delayed because symptoms either don't occur at all in the early stages of HH or consist of vague feelings of fatigue or lack of energy.

I go for a physical every year because my father died of heart trouble when I was 3 years old, and my mother died of cancer—I don't know what kind of cancer—when I was 12.

About six years ago, something came up with my iron count. My doctor said I had the iron count of a 90-year-old man. And the fact that I was still menstruating, which is when you should lose iron in the blood, was a red flag.

My doctor referred me to a gastroenterologist who monitored me and said it looked like I had hemochromatosis. I just panicked. Is this life-

threatening? Will it incapacitate me? It scared me because of my parents dying. It's my biggest fear—dropping dead early.

JUDY

Judy had no symptoms of HH. Fortunately, she scheduled yearly medical examinations, and her doctor included a blood test for iron, which detected high iron levels. With periodic phlebotomy her body iron stores will become normal and she will avoid organ damage from iron overload.

Judy's experience underscores the observation that women are relatively protected from excessive iron overload, compared to men, because they lose blood and iron via menstruation. As a result, in untreated cases, organ dysfunction due to iron accumulation typically occurs a decade later in women.

Two phases characterize the symptomatic stage of hemochromatosis: an early phase with nonspecific constitutional complaints, such as fatigue, and a later phase with symptoms related to organ dysfunction. Many people report fatigue as one of their earliest symptoms. Other symptoms can include lack of energy, lethargy, weakness, apathy, weight loss, aching of muscles and joints, or nonspecific abdominal discomforts. None of these symptoms is unique, specific, or diagnostic of hemochromatosis.

As stores of iron increase, later symptoms appear that reflect damage to specific organs. Iron deposits in the skin may cause a bronze tone. It's not unusual for people with hemochromatosis to look suntanned all year round. Liver disease can lead to swelling of the ankles or abdomen, a tendency to bruise or bleed, yellowing of the whites of the eyes, poor concentrating ability, memory lapses, or periods of confusion. Cardiac involvement might be signaled by buildup of fluid in the lungs or in the rest of the body and irregularity in heart rhythm. When HH involves the pancreas, diabetes mellitus may occur. Arthritis may be the first indicator of hemochromatosis, and sexual dysfunction and impotence are common.

Diagnosis is often delayed. A routine battery of lab tests usually doesn't include blood tests for excess iron. And even when the tests are included, the results may not be interpreted correctly. In a CDC-sponsored survey published in 1999, 2,851 patients reported via questionnaire that 67 percent were diagnosed first with arthritis, liver/gallbladder disease, stomach disorders, hormonal deficiencies, psychiatric problems, or diabetes before being diagnosed much later with hemochromatosis.

When I turned 34, I spent the next four years not feeling good at all. The doctors kept telling me I had an ulcer. If I ate, I got sick. If I didn't eat, I got sick. Then they tested my gallbladder. "Everything is fine," they'd say.

But it wasn't fine. After work, I'd go right to bed. I threw up bile and had terrible headaches. I slept the whole weekend. When I'd try to eat a bowl of cereal, I was too exhausted to get the spoon to my mouth.

My family doctor thought it was all in my head. Another doctor took out my appendix when I complained about my constant pain. And when I woke up after the operation, my first thought was that my pain wasn't near that scar at all. It was higher, closer to my rib cage.

Finally, I went to a doctor who said, "I know something is wrong, but I don't know what it is." He was the first to say that to me, and he sent me to a gastroenterologist who is my hero to this day. The gastroenterologist took a blood test and checked my ferritin (a protein that stores iron) level. No one had ever done that before. A ferritin level should be between 15 and 50. Mine was at 4,000!

STACY

Hemochromatosis produces multiple nonspecific symptoms that can lead physicians astray and delay diagnosis. For example, if your lab tests show high blood sugar, your primary physician might treat you for diabetes or refer you to an endocrinologist, a doctor who specializes in treating diabetes and other hormonal conditions. The dramatically obvious piece of the puzzle, diabetes, gets treated and you improve temporarily, but the root cause, hemochromatosis, remains undetected. You might feel better for a while, but inevitably you will feel sick again.

For some people, HH progresses more rapidly, and we don't know exactly why. However, in the case of liver disease the excessive use of alcohol, or other conditions such as viral hepatitis, accelerate progression.

My dad was diagnosed with hemochromatosis in 1985. He called my brother and me and said, "You need to get an iron test right away." It turned out that I didn't have elevated levels. But in 1994, I found out I had hepatitis C. At first I was too scared to have a liver biopsy, but I finally did. I told the doctors to check for HH at the same time. I wound up being okay on both counts—no damage.

Then I got pregnant. I never thought about what would happen when I stopped menstruating. I was less than three months pregnant, but my iron went way up. A biopsy showed that I had gone from no liver damage to stage 3. And I'm going, "What happened to stage 2?"

I had never paid much attention to HH. I discounted it, but in combination with hepatitis C, it can really aggravate it—like a double whammy!

BONNIE

Although it would be ideal if primary physicians were on the alert for hemochromatosis, this isn't always the case. Even doctors who are especially trained to diagnose HH, such as gastroenterologists, hepatologists, and hematologists, may miss the diagnosis. Gastroenterologists specialize in treating problems of digestive organs. Hepatologists are gastroenterologists who specifically treat liver diseases, and hematologists are specialists in blood disorders.

The Discovery of Hemochromatosis

In 1865, a French doctor, Armand Trousseau, described the syndrome of diabetes, cirrhosis of the liver, and bronze skin color. He later called this condition "bronze diabetes." In 1889, the famous German pathologist, H. von Recklinghausen, used the term "hemochromatosis" for the syndrome and concluded that iron was responsible for the characteristic pigmentation.

Joseph H. Sheldon, a British physician, collected the 311 case records that had appeared in medical literature since Trousseau's first description. In a 340-page monograph published in 1935, Sheldon pulled together a number of conflicting views. He replaced them with one unifying hypothesis that a single disease was responsible for affecting the many organs involved, that it was caused by "an inborn error of metabolism"[1] (an idea he first proposed in 1927), and that family studies suggested a hereditary pattern,

"Indeed," said Sheldon, "the relation of iron to the cells in hæmochromatosis appears to be on all fours with that of the lobster to the lobster pot—easy to get in but supremely difficult to get out."[2]

Over the years, researchers learned more about iron overload. They were able to measure the normal range of iron excretion and absorption with radioisotopes, determine that excess stored iron could be removed by phlebotomy, and explain that hemochromatosis was rarer in women because females normally lost blood (and, therefore, extra iron) during menstruation and pregnancies.

Family studies suggested inheritance patterns. Although scientists disagreed over exactly how the condition passed from generation to generation, the search for the hemochromatosis gene was on. In 1976, Simon and colleagues published their evidence that the iron-loading gene was associated with the HLA locus on chromosome 6. Meanwhile, with the advent of human leucocyte antigen (HLA) tissue typing and liver biopsy procedures, scientists conducted more studies investigating frequency and inheritance patterns.

In 1996, the breakthrough occurred. J. N. Feder, A. Gnirke, W. Thomas, Z. Tsuchihashi, and associates published their discovery of the HFE gene and two of its mutations, C282Y and H63D, which are linked to hemochromatosis. In the future, scientists expect to find more mutations.

Understanding Hemochromatosis

When von Recklinghausen named hemochromatosis in 1889, he described the "disease" he observed using Greek words. Hemo (or haemo, as von Recklinghausen spelled it) means blood, chroma means color (due to the copper or bronze-colored skin pigmentation), and osis comes from the Greek suffix for condition or disorder.

The underlying problem in hemochromatosis is excessive intestinal absorption of iron from the diet. Analysis of the components of a normal diet indicates that each 1000 calories of consumed food contains approximately 6 milligrams of iron. Normally, about 5 to 10 percent of this dietary iron is absorbed. The mutation in the HFE gene increases iron absorption by two- to three-fold.

The increase in iron absorption would not be harmful if it were balanced by an increase in elimination of iron from the body. Normally iron is removed from the body by the sloughing of cells from the lining of the intestine or skin, menstruation, or minor loss of blood through breaks in the skin or gastrointestinal tract. All of these mechanisms for removal of iron from the body operate at normal levels in patients with hemochromatosis. Because iron absorption is increased two- to three-fold but iron removal is not increased, iron accumulates in the body.

Most materials on hemochromatosis focus on the clinical or medical problems that arise from the excess accumulation of iron. But the person with hemochromatosis may experience other difficulties. Perhaps you have set off the metal detector at the airport, even after removing all metal watches and belts, because of the iron in your body. Or maybe friends have expressed envy about your nice tan that seems to last all winter long.

WHAT IS IRON? Iron is a metallic element. It is not a heavy metal, such as lead or gold, but a nutrient that all plants, animals, and humans must have to live. We need iron to make DNA (see next section). We also require iron for life-giving processes, such as creating hemoglobin to deliver oxygen throughout our bodies. (For a discussion of various forms of iron and how these forms exist in nature and in our bodies, see Chapter 6.) People normally get enough iron through their daily diets, but too much iron can harm you.

WHAT IS A GENETIC MUTATION? Many diseases or conditions are caused or programmed by mutations in the body's own genes.

In the center of each cell in your body are 46 threadlike chromosomes (23 pairs) that contain the genes that make you a unique human being. Genes are pairs of chemical codes that program the way your cells develop. They are made from a chemical called deoxyribonucleic acid (DNA). If you took the coiled strand of DNA from the chromosomes of just one of your cells and stretched it out, it would measure about six feet and contain more than 100,000 genes. We transmit our DNA, our individual genetic code, to our children via the DNA in our sperm and eggs. Each parent contributes half of the pair of each gene.

When a cell divides, the DNA copies itself. Sometimes, a mistake occurs in this copying process. This mistake, called a mutation, can cause a defect in the body's metabolism. (Metabolism is a term that refers to our body processes, including a whole host of chemical reactions that are necessary to sustain function and maintain life.) The mutation is then encoded in the DNA and passed on to future generations.

In hemochromatosis, the mutations tend to occur on chromosome 6 in the HFE gene, which determines how much iron your body absorbs. The mutations signal your body to absorb and store much more iron than you need, and the excess iron eventually can interfere with the way your organs function.

WHO HAS HEMOCHROMATOSIS? Hemochromatosis is defined as having excess iron stored in the body, leading to organ damage. Typically, the only people who develop this condition are those who have two gene mutations. Because you receive one gene from each parent, you may get two mutated genes (HH), one mutated gene and one normal gene (carrier), or two normal genes. If you inherit a pair of two mutated genes, you will probably show signs of hemochromatosis.

WHO IS A CARRIER? If you inherit one mutated gene and one normal gene, we call you a carrier, a person who may carry or transmit the gene for hemochromatosis. Scientists used to think that a carrier showed no signs of hemochromatosis, but we now know that some carriers may develop mild or modest iron overload. Typically the degree of overload in carriers is not sufficient to cause symptoms or organ damage. Genetic testing is the only reliable way to determine whether you have hemochromatosis or are a carrier.

Hemochromatosis is one of the most common of the thousands of genetic defects of metabolism that can occur. Unlike some genetic defects, such as cystic fibrosis, the damaging effects of hemochromatosis are preventable and treatable when detected early. (See Chapter 3 for a more detailed explanation of the genetics of HH.)

> *My grandfather died of bronze diabetes and heart complications in the 1940s when no one knew these were symptoms of hemochromatosis. How lucky I am to live now and not a hundred years ago.*
>
> *Now we can treat HH with phlebotomies. I'm grateful. The only time I whine is when the lab tech doesn't get the vein on the first poke—but that's minor.*
>
> CATHY

Other Conditions of Iron Overload (Not Hemochromatosis)

The focus of our book is hereditary hemochromatosis, and the vast majority of these cases are related to mutations in the HFE gene. However, a small subgroup of cases of hereditary hemochromatosis may be due to other mutations in the HFE gene not linked to the HLA locus on chromosome 6. Scientists are still investigating the genetic basis of these forms of hereditary hemochromatosis.

Iron overload also can occur in several other conditions. Patients with severe anemia may require multiple transfusions of blood over several years; iron accumulates with the breakdown of this transfused blood.

In unusual circumstances, an excessive intake of iron can lead to accumulation. One condition, African iron overload, may be related to excess intake of iron by drinking beer brewed in non-galvanized steel drums, coupled with increased intestinal absorption due to an as yet undefined iron-loading gene.

Patients with chronic liver diseases, such as alcoholic cirrhosis, fatty liver, and advanced viral hepatitis, may exhibit iron accumulation. In addition, a number of unusual genetic disorders are characterized by iron overload, including neonatal hemochromatosis, juvenile hemochromatosis, aceruloplasminemia, congenital atransferrinemia, Melanesian iron overload, and hyperferritinemia. The basis for iron overload in most of the latter conditions remains unknown.

Physicians caring for patients with alcoholic liver disease and chronic hepatitis C may also need to screen for hemochromatosis in patients with elevated iron studies. Both hemochromatosis and the carrier state for hemochromatosis have been associated with more aggressive disease in these patient populations.

Hemochromatosis: Early Detection Is the Key

In the remainder of this book we discuss in detail many issues of paramount importance to the patient and family dealing with hemochromatosis. As you read this book, remember one key point. Early detection and phlebotomy can avoid clinical complications.

We physicians, patients and families should be thankful for the medical technology that has provided us with the tools to insure early detection and appropriate therapy. HH is a preventable or curable condition. Undoubtedly, we are on the threshold of additional advances in our understanding of hemochromatosis and related disorders.

As a doctor, I'm happy when a patient is diagnosed early and together we can prevent the long-term complications of hemochromatosis. Patients who are diagnosed after complications arise may still have other victories along the way. Any disorder, especially a chronic one, tests a person's limits. My hope is that the following chapters will help you learn more about hemochromatosis and make you more comfortable with your choices and challenges from day to day.

> *Ay me! What perils do environ*
> *The man that meddles with cold iron!*
> SAMUEL BUTLER
> *Hudibras, Part I, Canto III*

REFERENCE

1. J. H. Sheldon, *Haemochromatosis* (London: Oxford University Press, 1935) 339.

2

WHEN YOU HAVE HEMOCHROMATOSIS

Blood Tests, Liver Biopsy, and Other Diagnostic Tests

After I had my tests for HH, my doctor said, "You have some high octane blood. There's lots of iron in it!"

LARRY

INTERPRETING RESULTS FROM DIAGNOSTIC TESTS can be confusing. Iron metabolism is complicated, and many conditions may affect iron levels. My patients often ask, "Why is my iron elevated? Are you sure I have hemochromatosis? Is my liver damaged? How accurate are these tests? Could the results be due to something else?

This chapter answers these questions and many others about the testing process for HH from the time you are diagnosed through the years of ongoing care (see Chapter 3 for information on genetic testing). It covers the following topics:

- *Diagnostic Tests for Hemochromatosis*
  TESTS FOR IRON
  SERUM IRON
  TOTAL IRON BINDING CAPACITY (TIBC) AND TRANSFERRIN
  SATURATION
  FERRITIN
  HLA TESTING
  GENE TESTING
  SUGGESTED ORDER OF DIAGNOSTIC TESTING
  LIVER IMAGING TESTS
    Ultrasonography (US, Ultrasound)
    Computed Tomography (CT Scan)
    Magnetic Resonance Imaging (MRI)
- *Liver Biopsy*
  PERCUTANEOUS BIOPSY PROCEDURE
  TRANSJUGULAR BIOPSY PROCEDURE
- *Interpreting Biopsy Results*
- *Liver Blood Tests*
  LIVER ENZYMES
  BILIRUBIN
  ALBUMIN
  CLOTTING FACTORS
  ALPHA-FETOPROTEIN
  COMPLETE BLOOD COUNT
  IRON STUDIES
- *Other Studies Related to Cardiac, Endocrine, and Joint Involvement*
  CARDIAC
    Echocardiogram
    Cardiac Catheterization and Endomyocardial Biopsy
  ENDOCRINE
    Tests for Diabetes Mellitus and Gonadal function
  JOINTS
    Radiologic Findings
    Needle Aspiration of Joint Fluid
- *Testing, Testing*

Diagnostic Tests for Hemochromatosis

TESTS FOR IRON. The average adult man without hemochromatosis has a total body iron content of approximately 35 to 45 milligrams per kilogram of body weight. Premenopausal women have lower stores due to periodic losses from menstruation (see Figure 2A).

Iron exists in several forms in the body. Two-thirds resides in the hemoglobin of red cells with each red cell containing approximately 1 billion atoms of iron. Most of the remaining iron exists in storage forms within liver cells, cells of the bone marrow, and other cells of the immune system called monocytes or macrophages. A special iron transport protein called transferrin, synthesized by the liver, circulates in the blood to shuttle iron from storage sites to other cells, such as bone marrow cells.

Iron stored inside cells accounts for approximately 1 gram of total body iron and is usually bound to proteins. Two-thirds of the stored iron is bound to ferritin, a protein that is metabolically active, soluble, and mobile inside the cell. One-third is bound to hemosiderin, an insoluble complex of aggregated ferritin and iron. Ferritin stores iron in cells and also circulates in the blood, but hemosiderin is typically large, relatively insoluble, and remains in tissues. In conditions of iron overload, the hemosiderin storage pool increases and accounts for "stainable iron" on tissue biopsies.

FIGURE 2A:
DISTRIBUTION OF IRON IN ADULTS[1]

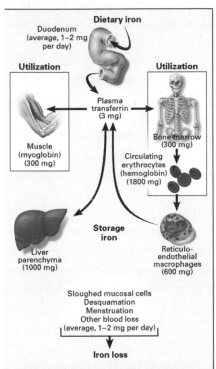

LEGEND 2A: *In otherwise normal individuals, the amount of iron taken in the diet is offset by loss of iron from the body from sloughing of cells from skin and gut, menstruation, and other blood loss. Most of the iron in the body is found in red blood cells and liver. Lesser amounts are found in muscle and other tissues.*

The principal abnormality of hemochromatosis, excessive intestinal iron absorption, leads to accumulation of iron within the body. Tests that measure the excess in total body iron are serum iron, total iron binding capacity (TIBC), transferrin saturation, and ferritin. The "gold standard" for determining the quantity of iron overload is the liver biopsy.

SERUM IRON. Serum iron concentration is a measure of circulating levels of iron. A poor marker of total body iron and level, serum iron can fluctuate nonspecifically in response to a change in diet, inflammation, liver injury, or use of supplemental iron. Serum iron, when used alone, is poorly predictive of either the presence or absence of hemochromatosis. Serum iron level must be interpreted in the context of its carrier protein, transferrin; it is not recommended as a single test for either screening or diagnosis for hemochromatosis.

TOTAL IRON BINDING CAPACITY (TIBC) AND TRANSFERRIN SATURATION. Transferrin is a relatively small protein of 77,000 kilodaltons (kD) molecular weight. It is the main transport protein for iron and the main determinant of total iron binding capacity in the blood. In normal individuals, TIBC is typically 300 to 350 micrograms (ug) of iron per deciliter of plasma; about one third of this capacity is saturated with iron, i.e, transferrin saturation equals 33 percent.

Several studies have indicated that transferrin saturation is a useful screening tool because nearly all adult patients with hemochromatosis will have an increased transferrin saturation. Useful cutoffs that increase the likelihood for hemochromatosis are saturation greater than 50 percent in premenopausal women and greater than 60 percent in men or postmenopausal women. Approximately 74 to 86 percent of patients with values exceeding these cutoffs will have hemochromatosis.

FERRITIN. Ferritin is a large protein of 480,000 kD molecular weight, serves as a storage depot for iron, and exists in both tissue and circulating forms. Chemical analysis suggests that as many as 4500 atoms of iron can be stored within a single ferritin molecule.

> *We had just had a baby so I applied for life insurance. When I went for the insurance test, I got denied because my liver enzymes were high. I thought it meant I had too much to drink the night before.*
>
> *My doctor checked me out, and I had a 6500 serum ferritin level. It took one-and-a-half years of phlebotomies to get it down. A liver biopsy found cirrhosis. I was 29 years old.*
>
> AL

Plasma ferritin concentrations correlate with total body iron stores and are typically elevated in patients with hemochromatosis. However, some patients with hemochromatosis have normal ferritin levels and, conversely, ferritin levels may increase in other conditions in response to inflammation.

These variations make ferritin imperfect as a screening tool when used alone. When used in screening, it is commonly combined with transferrin saturation. Because ferritin typically correlates with total body iron, it is frequently used to monitor the effectiveness of phlebotomy in reducing iron stores. In patients with confirmed hereditary hemochromatosis, ferritin greater than 1000 nanograms per milliliter (ng/ml) correlates with significant hepatic fibrosis or cirrhosis.

HLA (HUMAN LEUKOCYTE ANTIGEN) TESTING. HLA testing is of historical importance, but is rarely, if ever, done for diagnostic purposes today. In 1975, Simon and colleagues demonstrated that the gene for hemochromatosis was in close proximity to genes for HLA-A and HLA-B on chromosome 6.

At that time there were no measurements for the hemochromatosis gene or its product, but there were methods for determining HLA types. Because the gene for hemochromatosis and HLA were in close physical proximity, transmission of hemochromatosis could be inferred by using the pattern of inheritance of specific HLA types. HLA typing could predict with reasonable certainty the likelihood of hemochromatosis in siblings of an affected individual. However, HLA typing had limited utility in clinical practice, and current gene tests have supplanted HLA for diagnostic purposes.

GENE TESTING. Approximately 90 percent of cases of hemochromatosis are due to one of two patterns of mutations in the HFE gene: two C282Y mutations (homozygous for C282Y) or one C282Y plus one H63D mutation (compound heterozygous). People with one isolated C282Y mutation, one isolated H63D mutation, or two H63D mutations, may exhibit mildly elevated iron tests but typically do not develop hemochromatosis.

Gene tests are highly specific and accurate but should be used in the context of other aspects of the evaluation. Despite the availability of gene testing, determining iron overload by blood tests and liver biopsy is still important because the degree of iron overload in patients homozygous for C282Y is highly variable, and others with iron overload may have negative tests for C282Y. Current results suggest that up to 10 percent of cases of severe iron overload may be due to as yet unidentified additional mutations. (See Chapter 3 for a complete description of genetic tests and their interpretation.)

SUGGESTED ORDER OF DIAGNOSTIC TESTING. Anthony Tavill, M.D., recently published the American Association for the Study of Liver Diseases (AASLD) practice guidelines for hemochromatosis. When an adult is suspected to have HH, the initial screening should include transferrin saturation and ferritin. If transferrin saturation is less than 45 percent and ferritin is normal, then hemochromatosis is unlikely and no further testing is warranted.

Exceptions could include young or premenopausal first-degree relatives of a documented case with hemochromatosis. In these circumstances, gene testing may be recommended, even if iron studies are normal. Gene testing is recommended for any patient with elevated transferrin saturation and ferritin. Most patients with high iron saturations also will require a liver biopsy to determine the amount of iron and the severity of fibrosis in the liver (see Liver Biopsy, below).

LIVER IMAGING TESTS. Doctors often order imaging tests of the liver to exclude biliary tract disease and mass lesions, such as liver cancer. The most commonly used tests are ultrasonography, CT (computed tomography), and MRI (magnetic resonance imaging). Each is unique and gives specific information.

Ultrasonography (US, Ultrasound). Ultrasonography is a safe and painless way to investigate the size, structure, and the vascular (blood) supply of the liver. It's commonly used in the initial assessment of the biliary system and for liver tumors.

With regular phlebotomies, my liver and spleen went back to normal size. My doctor says my chance of getting liver cancer is greater than the average person, so he does an ultrasound every year. A couple of years ago, he found a spot. When he did a CT scan, it turned out to be a hematoma (bruise).

AMY

Ultrasonic waves penetrate the body tissues and a recording device picks up reflected sound waves that yield an image of the liver. You can compare it to exploring for oil by using seismographic recordings of the earth's formations.

Ultrasound helps determine liver size and texture and the size of bile ducts and blood vessels. Doppler probes added to ultrasound can detect direction and rates of blood flow in vessels going to and from the liver. Your physician may order ultrasound to pinpoint the liver's location just before a biopsy.

Computed Tomography (CT Scan). Unlike ultrasound, computed tomography (CT scan) uses a highly sophisticated X-ray machine to scan the internal organs with minimal radiation. CT scans are used to confirm the findings of ultrasound and to get a clearer view because, unlike ultrasound, CT scans aren't blocked by air in the bowel. The scans are also more standardized and much less dependent on the expertise of the technician performing the test.

I never had a CT scan before. It made all kinds of noise. That would be hard if you're claustrophobic, but I'm not. Turned out my heart's good, and my kidneys are all right.

I didn't feel claustrophobic during the CT scan because I wasn't fully in the tube. It passes over you three to four times. You have to plan a half a day. You have to get there early, drink a fluid, and wait. It cost me $2,500, but my insurance covered it.

CT scans define the size and texture of the liver and can detect an early liver tumor. Some studies suggest that CT scans can also detect iron accumulations in the liver when the iron concentration in the tissue is very high.

Magnetic Resonance Imaging (MRI). Unlike ultrasound and CT scans, MRI measures special signals (see Figure 2B) from the body's water molecules. Images are created from these signals. Magnetic resonance imaging is used mainly to diagnose liver cancers and is particularly sensitive in detecting cancers in patients with hemochromatosis. Some studies suggest that MRI can also detect iron accumulations in the liver

FIGURE 2B:
MRI (MAGNETIC RESONANCE IMAGING) SCANS OF AN UNAFFECTED INDIVIDUAL
(LEFT) AND A PATIENT WITH CIRRHOSIS DUE TO HEMOCHROMATOSIS (RIGHT)

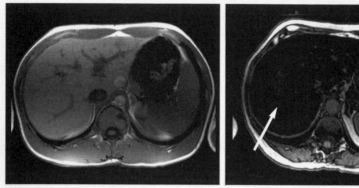

NORMAL LIVER   CIRHHOTIC LIVER

LEGEND 2B: *The liver of an unaffected individual is shown on the left. The liver from the patient with hemochromatosis has a black appearance on MRI (white arrow) due to the trapping of the magnetic signals by the markedly increased concentration of iron in the liver. The spleen (Sp) was enlarged due to cirrhosis of the liver.*

when the iron concentration in the tissue is very high. Neither CT scans nor MRI are sufficiently precise to replace liver biopsy in accurately determining the amount of iron in the liver.

Liver Biopsy

As I stated before, a liver biopsy is the "gold standard" for measuring iron overload and is useful in determining the extent of liver damage and fibrosis. A biopsy should be considered when a suspected individual has either elevated blood tests for iron or tests positive on genetic analysis.

An exception to the requirement for a biopsy might be the relatively young patient (under 40 years old), with two mutations for C282Y (homozygote), ferritin less than 1000, and normal liver tests. Elevated iron studies and gene testing clinch the diagnosis of hereditary hemochromatosis. In addition, a relatively young age, coupled with normal liver tests and only modest elevation in ferritin, virtually excludes the possibility of cirrhosis. This patient could undergo therapeutic phlebotomy without a biopsy.

Just the word "biopsy" makes people apprehensive, but it's an essential test to determine the amount of iron and the extent of liver damage (see Figure 2C). Only a biopsy can give your doctor a true idea of the condition of your liver. You need a biopsy for three main reasons:

- *It confirms the diagnosis and rules out other disorders, such as alcoholic liver disease, viral hepatitis, granulomatous liver disease, infections, or biliary tract disorders.*
- *It quantifies the amount of iron.*
- *It establishes the degree of scarring and whether cirrhosis is present.*

FIGURE 2C:
LIVER BIOPSIES STAINED FOR IRON

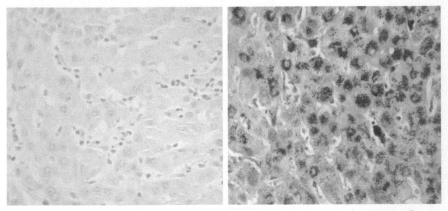

LEGEND 2C: *A normal liver is shown on the left. In comparison, the biopsy from a patient with hemochromatosis (right) demonstrates dark, dense, black granules within the liver cells and other cells of the liver. Iron granules are intensely blue when stained with Prussian blue.*

Biopsies may be done over many years to record the progression. Once cirrhosis has developed, there is little reason to continue the biopsies.

PERCUTANEOUS BIOPSY PROCEDURE. Percutaneous means that the biopsy needle passes through the skin (typically on the right side of the abdomen). Years ago, liver biopsies were often performed under general anesthesia and required a short hospital stay. Today it's an outpatient procedure that literally takes seconds. In fact, you'll spend most of your time getting ready for the biopsy.

The average biopsy is very small, varying between 1 to 3 centimeters in length and .5 to 2 millimeters in diameter. This amount of tissue represents only 0.002 percent of your total liver.

A biopsy is invasive, however, and you will be asked to sign an informed consent form. It's a good idea to select a doctor who frequently performs this procedure and is very familiar with it. Studies have suggested that the complication rate is lower when physicians perform the procedure more than 50 times a year.

I was terrified to have a liver biopsy. First they did an MRI to locate my liver. The biopsy was like someone takes a fist and gives you the hardest punch to your chest. They went in two times.

The doctor called me to tell me I had no cirrhosis of the liver, no damage. But I'd have to be phlebotomized until they got my hemotocrit and hemoglobin count down to less than 10/30.

For my liver biopsy, they used ultrasound to locate the lung and liver—to make sure they missed the lung. Then they used a marker to make a target on my rib cage. The only thing I felt was when the doctor marked my skin with a pen. I heard two clicks, and then he said, "We're done."

The liver biopsy was relatively easy. The part that wasn't explained to me was that when they go through the rib cage, they sometimes hit the nerve to the shoulder. So within two hours of the biopsy, I had a pain in my shoulder. They explained that everyone is different.

It's helpful to plan a quiet, restful period after a biopsy. In my experience, most patients' fears come from not knowing what to expect. Here's how the procedure goes:

Your physician examines you carefully to decide exactly where to place the biopsy needle and cleanses the skin with iodine or an antiseptic solution. Then you'll get a local anesthetic, as you do at the dentist's, at the spot where the biopsy needle will be placed. Some doctors also prescribe intravenous benzodiazepine with a narcotic to lessen anxiety and discomfort.

You'll feel strong pressure when the needle is inserted, but the whole procedure takes only a few seconds for a small core of tissue to be obtained. Then you'll be rolled onto your right side to help control any bleeding from the surface of the liver. You'll stay in the procedure area for two to four hours for observation. If you're stable, with no symptoms, you'll be discharged. Otherwise, you may be admitted to the hospital for observation.

After performing biopsies on hundreds of patients, I've seen very few complications. Reported rates of complications vary from 0.1 to 3 percent. As many as 1 to 3 percent of patients undergoing liver biopsy are hospitalized for complications after the procedure, mainly for pain or low blood pressure. If bleeding from the surface of the liver occurs, the patient may require transfusions or even an operation. In rare cases, the biopsy needle may pierce another organ, such as the bowel, gallbladder, kidney, or lung. Death occurs very rarely, with reported rates varying between 1 in 10,000 to 1 in 12,000 biopsies.

TRANSJUGULAR BIOPSY PROCEDURE. A radiologist passes a catheter through a neck vein into the liver and takes a biopsy sample. This technique minimizes bleeding because it avoids puncturing the liver capsule. Tissue samples obtained with this procedure are generally smaller than samples from the percutaneous technique. This type of biopsy is often performed in the "high-risk" patient (with cirrhosis or other underlying clotting disorders) and, therefore, reported complication rates are higher. Reported complication rates vary from 1.3 to 20.2 percent, and death occurs between 1 in 200 to 1 in 1000 biopsies.

Interpreting Biopsy Results

I was working on a government site where we were required to take physical exams every year because of the contaminants. A new doctor included iron in the heavy metal screening. I got a letter saying my iron levels were high. It was the first time I heard the word hemochromatosis.

A liver biopsy showed that I had 20 to 30 times the normal amount of iron in my liver—a huge amount. They did a Prussian blue stain. My liver was at stage 3+ on the fibrosis scale.

BERNIE

Your doctor will tell you the results of your biopsy in terms of histologic stages. Histology means the examination of tissue under the microscope. There are five histologic stages of scarring of the liver:

- STAGE 0 *is characterized by lack of any increase in scar tissue.*
- STAGE I *is characterized by a minimal increase in the normal amount of scar tissue.*
- STAGE II *features early scarring (fibrosis) in one zone (portal)*

of the liver.
- STAGE III *shows bridging of the fibrosis between adjacent portal tracts.*
- STAGE IV *is cirrhosis (advanced scarring with loss of normal liver architecture).*

Histologic stages don't correspond very well to either symptoms or signs of liver disease, and the rate of progression is variable. For example, a patient with slowly progressive fibrosis may maintain an early histologic stage for many years or even decades. Another patient may progress to cirrhosis more rapidly. The stages of liver fibrosis overlap but are distinguishable under the microscope.

Liver Blood Tests

Life with hemachromatosis means lots of blood tests to monitor your condition. Have you ever wondered what the numbers really mean? Read the next few pages to review and understand the warning signals of six basic blood tests:

- *Liver enzymes*
- *Bilirubin*
- *Albumin*
- *Clotting factors*
- *Complete blood count*
- *Iron studies*

Doctors frequently test blood in hemachromatosis patients because blood tests warn of changes. The most informative tests "dip" into the bloodstream to measure liver injury (enzymes) or assess liver function (bilirubin, albumin, clotting factors, complete blood count). At first, you may feel intimidated by medical terminology, acronyms, and numbers, but learning about these basic tests will help you understand your doctor's interpretation of results (see Table 2A).

LIVER ENZYMES. A liver cell produces proteins, called enzymes, that live within the cell or its membranes. In a way, you can think of your liver as a powerful chemical factory; it changes raw materials into the substances your body needs. Enzymes are catalysts that help a liver cell

TABLE 2A: NORMAL AND ABNORMAL VALUES FOR LABORATORY TESTS

TEST	NORMAL RANGE	ABNORMAL RANGE MILD TO MODERATE	SEVERE
LIVER ENZYMES			
AST	<40 IU/L	40–200	>200
ALT	<40 IU/L	40–200	>200
GGT	<60 IU/L	60–200	>200
ALKALINE PHOSPHATASE	<112 IU/L	112–300	>300
LIVER FUNCTION TESTS			
BILIRUBIN	<1.2 MG/DL	1.2–2.5	>2.5
ALBUMIN	3.5–4.5 G/DL	3.0–3.5	<3.0
PROTHROMBIN TIME	<14 SECONDS	14-17	>17
BLOOD COUNT			
WBC	>6000	3000–6000	<3000
HCT	>40	35–40	<35
PLATELETS	>150,000	100,000–150,000	<100,000

KEY:
IU = *International Units*   **L** = liter
dl = deciliter   **mg** = milligrams
AST(SGOT) = aspartate aminotransferase   **ALT** (SGPT) = alanine aminotransferase
GGT = gamma-glutamyl transferase   **WBC** = white blood count
HCT = hematocrit (% of blood occupied by red blood cells)

do its job of creating the specific chemical changes that give your body fuel to live. Here are the names of the enzymes you need to remember:

- *ALT (SGPT)—alanine aminotransferase*
- *AST (SGOT)—aspartate aminotransferase*
- *GGT—gamma-glutamyl transferase*
- *alkaline phosphatase*

By measuring their level in your blood, doctors can monitor ongoing liver injury. Why? Under normal conditions, the level of these enzymes in your bloodstream is relatively low. But when liver cells are injured, destroyed, or die, the cell becomes leaky, and the enzymes escape into the blood that's circulating through the liver. When the cell is injured, liver enzyme levels in the blood rise.

What do the numbers mean? Table 2A shows normal and abnormal test values. Blood test patterns relate somewhat to the type of liver injury. Typical hemochromatosis patients show increases in ALT and AST and lesser increases in GGT and alkaline phosphatase. Those with cirrhosis or who have an underlying disorder of the biliary tract (the ducts that drain bile from the liver into the intestine) may have modest elevations in GGT and alkaline phosphatase. In some unusual cases of hemochromatosis, I have even seen a predominant elevation in GGT.

Patients tend to focus on their ALT and AST counts, but other tests are more important in measuring the health of your liver.

BILIRUBIN. When red blood cells complete their life cycle and break down naturally in your body, they produce a yellow pigment that's passed to the liver and excreted into bile. Bile helps your body digest food, but the pigment, which has no digestive function, is called bilirubin. Blood levels of bilirubin tend to fluctuate in patients with hepatitis, although a prolonged persistent elevation in bilirubin usually means severe liver dysfunction and possibly cirrhosis.

Here's why. Most of the time, the body produces as many red blood cells as it breaks down, so you produce a constant amount of bilirubin. However, if your blood cells break down more rapidly (hemolysis) or your liver function becomes impaired, the bilirubin levels in your blood rise.

Your liver has to go to work to take up the excess bilirubin into the liver cell, metabolize it to make it more water-soluble for excretion into bile, and send it through special passages and ducts into the intestine. Microbes in the gut continue to metabolize the bilirubin until you expel it. (Stercobilin, a brown pigment derived from bilirubin, creates the dark brown color of feces.)

When the liver fails to eliminate bilirubin from the blood, the skin and whites of the eyes turn yellow (jaundice), urine darkens, and the color of the bowel movement lightens. In case you've wondered, now you know why your doctor asks you probing questions about the color of your feces.

ALBUMIN. Albumin is another protein synthesized (manufactured) by the liver. Liver cells secrete albumin to maintain the volume of blood in arteries and veins. When albumin levels drop to extremely low levels, fluid may leak out of the blood vessels into the surrounding tissues. This causes swelling, known as edema. Normal albumin levels range between 3.5 to 4.5 grams/deciliter. Usually, edema occurs when levels drop below 2.5 grams/deciliter.

Unlike liver enzyme increases, which occur within hours to days of the liver injury, albumin levels don't fall unless there has been chronic progressive liver injury for at least one month or more. This is because albumin has a long residence time in the plasma; its half-life is approximately 30 days. A decrease in serum albumin, therefore, reflects a slowly progressive, ongoing reduction in the liver's ability to synthesize this protein.

Be aware that there are non-liver reasons for albumin to decrease and your physician will take these into account when interpreting test results. Nonetheless, a significant sustained decrease in serum albumin may mean poor liver function and cirrhosis of the liver.

CLOTTING FACTORS. Remember our comparison of the liver to a chemical factory? The liver also synthesizes many proteins that maintain normal blood clotting. Prothrombin time (PT) is the name of the most common test that measures a combination of blood clotting factors. If your prothrombin time increases, it means your liver isn't creating enough factors, so it takes your blood longer to clot.

Unlike albumin, clotting factors can decrease rapidly—within days, or even hours, of a severe liver injury. In severe cases, clotting disturbances may signal the need for an early transplant. In patients with hemochromatosis and chronic liver disease, a prolonged prothrombin time can be a warning that the liver is having trouble with its synthetic functions.

Typically, doctors will administer vitamin K, a vitamin essential for normal clotting factors, to determine whether the clotting disorder is reversible. Patients who have persistent, prolonged elevations in prothrombin time that don't respond to vitamin K may need to be considered for liver transplantation.

ALPHA-FETOPROTEIN. This is a protein that regenerative cells or cancer cells secrete into blood. Increased blood levels of alpha-fetoprotein may indicate the development of liver cancer (see Chapter 10).

COMPLETE BLOOD COUNT. The complete blood count test can be a detection system for liver scarring. Blood from your spleen flows through your liver via the portal vein. When the liver becomes scarred, it creates resistance to this blood flow (called portal hypertension), and the blood may back up into the spleen. When this happens, the spleen enlarges and traps blood elements, removing them from circulation and lowering blood counts.

Although all components of the blood count may decrease, those most sensitive to this condition are the white blood cell and platelet counts. Patients with portal hypertension from cirrhosis of the liver often have low counts. Similarly, patients may have an enlarged spleen, resulting from severe cirrhotic disease, and may need to be considered for liver transplantation.

IRON STUDIES. Serum transferrin saturation and ferritin are often measured to track body iron studies over time—most commonly when people are undergoing therapeutic phlebotomy (see Chapters 5 and 9).

Other Studies Related to Cardiac, Endocrine, and Joint Involvement

CARDIAC. Iron deposits in the heart typically interfere with normal heart function, impairing the ability to contract and causing fluid buildup in the body. Three main tests assess cardiac hemochromatosis: echocardiography, cardiac catheterization, and endomyocardial biopsy.

Echocardiogram. Echocardiography uses ultrasound to image the heart and measure its contractile activity. Noninvasive and useful in measuring the pump function of the heart, echocardiography can be used to measure the effects of phlebotomy and other treatments on cardiac function. Echocardiography is also effective in imaging heart valves and their function; it can be used to define impairment in heart muscle function that could signal significant underlying coronary artery disease.

Cardiac Catheterization and Endomyocardial Biopsy. Many patients with hemochromatosis who have cardiac dysfunction may have another underlying cause such as valvular or coronary artery disease. When this is suspected or when measurement of cardiac iron content is warranted, it may be necessary to perform heart catheterization. Evaluation of the coronary arteries requires arterial catheterization, usually in the femoral artery (main artery in the groin), but performance of endomyocardial biopsy is typically done in the right ventricle and only requires venous catheterization.

ENDOCRINE: TESTS FOR DIABETES MELLITUS AND GONADAL FUNCTION. The most common endocrine disorder, diabetes mellitus, is typically diagnosed from routine studies of blood or urine. Blood tests are also used for assessment of gonadal and reproductive function.

JOINTS. Chronic arthritis involving the second and third joints between the hand and fingers is typical of hemochromatosis. These joints are called metacarpal (hand)–phalangeal (finger) joints.

Radiologic Findings. Plain radiographs may show distinctive patterns that may point to the diagnosis. Features that strongly suggest hemochromatosis are narrowing of joint spaces, loss of cartilage, bone cyst formation, and bone loss at the top of the metacarpal bones. In addition, the metacarpal bones may be squared with hooked, boney spurs, and cartilage calcifications are often present.

Needle Aspiration of Joint Fluid. Rarely, fluid in a swollen joint is removed (aspirated with a needle). The fluid is typically clear without much inflammation but contains crystals of calcium.

Testing, Testing

In the past few years, I've seen the advancement of specific new tests that help monitor your health. But all too often I find that patients feel shut out by the complicated language of test results. Don't worry if you didn't absorb every detail. Use these pages as a reference guide.

Ask for copies of your tests. When you have questions, look up the explanations in these pages. Often, your physician can calm your fears if you voice them. Talk with your doctor.

> *If gold ruste, what shal iren do?*
> CHAUCER
> *The Canterbury Tales*

REFERENCE

1. Nancy C. Andrews. "Disorders of Iron Metabolism." *New England Journal of Medicine* 341; 26(1999): 1986.

3

GENETIC TESTS

What Do They Mean?

You don't hear much about hemochromatosis, and so many people can have it. My husband and I were tested, and he is homozygous. Now each of my kids has one mutated gene. What if they marry someone else with the mutation?

I can't get my kids to have their spouses checked. They tell me I worry too much. But people don't have to suffer if they catch HH in time.

JANET

W E LIVE AT THE DAWN OF A NEW ERA IN MEDICAL biotechnology, the cracking of the human genetic code. In 1988, scientists began to map every gene in the human body in a study called the Human Genome Project. Currently, more than 100,000 human genes have been defined. This is an exciting and hopeful time for people with hereditary conditions, such as hemochromatosis.

Imagine the intricate work involved in mapping the HH gene. First, researchers had to figure out which chromosome to map—chromosome 6. Then they had to record the precise order of thousands of pairs of genes until they located the HFE gene and its mutations involved in hemochromatosis.

Note: Guidelines for gene testing continue to evolve. Gene tests and iron tests complement each other; your physician will interpret the results of gene tests in the context of iron studies. I typically don't recommend gene testing until my patient is an adult and can weigh the pros and cons.

As with all technological advances, discoveries raise new ethical questions. For example, gene testing offers important—even lifesaving—information, but will this information affect your privacy, medical records, or insurance? In this chapter, we will review some basic facts about genetics, the hemochromatosis gene mutations, and the procedures and ethical/social issues involved in gene testing.

- *You and Your Genes: An Introduction*
  - ORGANS, TISSUES, CELLS
  - CHROMOSOMES
  - DNA AND GENES
  - WHAT DO GENES HAVE TO DO WITH
    - HEMOCHROMATOSIS?
  - RNA AND PROTEINS
- *The HFE Gene*
  - MUTATIONS CAUSING HEMOCHROMATOSIS: C282Y,
    - H63D, OTHER
  - TRANSMISSION OF HEMOCHROMATOSIS MUTATION
    - IN FAMILIES
  - HETEROZYGOTE
  - HOMOZYGOTE
  - COMPOUND HETEROZYGOTE
- *Genetic Testing*
  - WHO SHOULD BE TESTED?
- *Genetic Counseling*
  - WHAT IS GENETIC COUNSELING?
  - FINDING AND SELECTING A GENETIC COUNSELOR
  - INTERPRETING THE RESULTS OF GENETIC (DNA) TESTS
  - CASE HISTORY
    - Reason for Request of Genetic Testing
    - Results of Additional Testing of the Family
    - Outcomes
- *Questions People Ask About Genetic Testing for Hemochromatosis*

You and Your Genes: An Introduction

ORGANS, TISSUES, CELLS. Background information about your body's structure and genetic machinery will help you understand the genetic nature of hemochromatosis. *(Note: Skip to "What Do Genes Have to Do with Hemochromatosis?" if you don't want to read this background material.)* Let's begin with a description of the body's largest entities, its systems.

A system is a group of organs that work together to perform a set of related functions. An organ is a grouping of cells and tissues in a system with its own set of well-defined functions. The liver, for example, is an organ that is part of the digestive system. (One of the liver's functions is to produce bile, which travels through the bile duct to the gastrointestinal tract, where it aids in digesting and absorbing nutrients, such as iron.) Tissues consist of cells and proteins that form the fibrous network of organs.

The primary building block of all tissues, organs, and systems, however, is the cell. Each cell contains programming for a specific "job." Bile duct cells, for example, aid in the secretion and transport of electrolytes and water.

Every cell has a plasma membrane, cytoplasm, and a nucleus. The plasma membrane encloses the cell. Unique proteins embedded in this membrane transport fluid, electrolytes, and other material across the membrane, while other proteins act as receptors to relay signals to the interior of the cell.

Inside the cell, the cytoplasm contains the machinery to perform most cell functions, including metabolism, synthesis, and secretion. The nucleus houses chromosomes, DNA, and genes with their regulatory elements.

CHROMOSOMES. Chromosomes are cellular structures that coordinate the distribution of DNA and genes during DNA reproduction (replication) and cell division. Each tightly organized chromosome contains the DNA for your genes and specific regulatory proteins to stabilize the DNA. Chromosomes are relatively large; you can view them with a standard laboratory microscope.

Each human cell has 23 pairs of chromosomes (for a total of 46). During cell division, the identical pairs duplicate the chromosomal makeup so that the two new cells they produce have genetic material identical to the original cell. This is true for most cells. When a liver cell (hepatocyte) replicates, for example, it divides to form two new cells with identical chromosomal and genetic constitution. That's why liver cells beget liver cells and not other organ cells.

However, not all cells divide in this fashion. The notable exceptions are sperm and egg (oocyte, ovary cell), where only one of the pair of chromosomes is maintained. Thus, when sperm and egg combine, the resulting cell has the full complement of chromosomes—one-half from the male sperm and one-half from the female egg.

In the transmission of hemochromatosis, you must inherit one HFE mutation via a chromosome from your mother and another HFE mutation via a chromosome from your father to get full-blown hereditary hemochromatosis. Carriers inherit a single HFE mutation from a chromosome from either their father or mother.

DNA AND GENES. DNA is the abbreviation for deoxyribonucleic acid, the large macromolecule that encrypts genetic information within its structure. Prior to the discovery of the double helix of DNA by Watson and Crick in 1953, the chemical nature of genes was attributed to proteins, RNA (ribonucleic acid), or other unknown cellular constituents. The discovery of the organizational framework of DNA set the course for investigations into the genetic makeup of cells and all living beings.

The structure of DNA determines its ability to encode information. The backbone of the molecule is a chain of sugar residues of deoxyribose bonded to each other via phosphate linkages. Each molecule of deoxyribose binds to one of four specific nucleoside molecules, called bases: adenine, guanine, thymine, and cytosine.

The double helix of DNA consists of two chains organized in a spiral connected to each other by the chemical interaction of the nucleoside bases. Adenine on one chain always binds to thymine on the other chain, and guanine on one chain always binds to cytosine on the other chain. Prior to cell division, DNA replicates by splitting the two chains, each of which forms a template for the formation of new DNA molecules. Exact replicas of each DNA molecule are made in this fashion.

Genes, segments of contiguous portions of DNA, provide the code for synthesis of specific proteins. The order and composition of bases in DNA determine the composition of amino acids that make up protein. Each triplicate of bases, called a codon, specifically encodes for a unique amino acid. A mutation is an event that only occurs in DNA and results in a change in a base pair.

You may encounter the term genotype. A genotype is the pattern of the inherited gene mutations, such as C282Y.

WHAT DO GENES HAVE TO DO WITH HEMOCHROMATOSIS? The HFE gene provides a code for synthesizing a specific protein involved with the regulation of iron absorption by the intestine. The C282Y mutation of the HFE gene substitutes guanine for adenine at position 845 of the HFE gene. This mutation changes the coding for the amino acids in the resultant protein from cysteine to tyrosine at position 282 of the protein. The effect of this mutation is to produce a new type of HFE protein which increases iron absorption and is less regulated by the buildup in total body iron.

RNA AND PROTEINS. RNA, ribonucleic acid, is similar to DNA in that it is a long chain macromolecule comprised of a sugar (ribose), phosphate, and nucleosides. It differs from DNA in that the sugar is ribose instead of deoxyribose, it is single stranded, and uracil substitutes for thymine as a nucleoside base. RNA is the intermediate between the genes in DNA and resulting proteins. The order of base pairs in messenger RNAs dictates the sequence of amino acids in proteins.

The nature and function of proteins is determined by the amino acid sequence and the conformational changes that occur in the protein after it is synthesized. For example, some proteins insert themselves into the plasma membrane and function as channels between the cell and external fluids, while other proteins are secreted into the blood to transport lipids such as fat or cholesterol. Still others may function as factors to prevent bleeding.

The key sequence to remember is:

DNA   Gene mutation occurs here.
↓
RNA   Receives message from gene to encode for protein.
↓
Protein Regulates iron absorption.

The HFE Gene

MUTATIONS CAUSING HEMOCHROMATOSIS. More than 90 percent of hemochromatosis cases are due to the inheritance of two of the C282Y mutations of the HFE gene (the vast majority of cases) or one C282Y mutation and one H63D mutation. Approximately 5 to 7 percent of cases are due to other unidentified mutations of non-HFE genes. There are well documented Italian families with iron overload, comparable to HFE-related HH, that lack both C282Y and H63D mutations and where the genetic abnormality is not localized to chromosome 6. The likelihood exists, therefore, that mutations of genes other than HFE may also cause hereditary hemochromatosis.

TRANSMISSION OF HFE MUTATIONS IN FAMILIES. As of this writing, only two mutations of the HFE gene have been associated with hereditary hemochromatosis: C282Y and H63D. Two C282Y mutations or one C282Y mutation plus one H63D mutation cause HH. Interestingly, two mutations of H63D do not cause HH. Therefore, to get HH you would need to receive one C282Y mutation from each of your parents or one C282Y mutation from one parent and one H63D mutation from the other.

HETEROZYGOTE. When an affected individual carries only a single mutation, we refer to that individual as a heterozygote. He or she received the abnormal gene from one parent. In some genetic disorders, receiving one abnormal gene is sufficient to cause disease, but in hemochromatosis, heterozygotes are often called carriers and typically lack symptoms of disease.

HOMOZYGOTE. A homozygote possesses two identical mutations of a single gene. The term homozygosity refers specifically to genetic makeup and does not necessarily imply iron overload or risk of hemochromatosis. For example, in the case of C282Y mutations, homozygosity is associated with HH, but in the case of H63D, homozygosity is not associated with HH.

COMPOUND HETEROZYGOTE. This term applies to the person who possesses two different mutations of a single gene. In the case of hemochromatosis, this typically refers to the patient who is positive for one C282Y mutation and one H63D mutation. Compound heterozygotes are at risk for iron overload and HH. This finding suggests that the H63D mutation, by itself, is incapable of causing iron overload but permits HH to develop in the presence of C282Y.

My dad died in 1996, and I think he died from hemochromatosis. He had a ferritin of 975 when I took him to my hematologist, plus he had pancreatic damage. We found out he was a compound heterozygote. His blood sugar was off the charts, and he was so fatigued.

We used to tease him all the time because he was a minister, and he would fall asleep whenever my grandmother played the organ. At the dinner table, his eyes would just slam shut.

There are days when my eyes slam shut, too. And my iron is not as high as my dad's.

The material I read is mostly about C282Y. There's always an asterisk that says they don't know about H63D, but I think we'll find out a lot more soon about compound heterozygotes like me. I think we tend to distribute iron differently. I've got these bronzy patches on my face, for example, that most people with HH don't have.

I was so anxious about my daughter until we tested her. She just has one H63D mutation—so that's good.

I was having a lot of symptoms: fatigue, and a lot of pain in the solar plexus. The pain was so bad that I panicked.

A hepatologist did a biopsy, and my liver was not saturated with iron. I didn't need treatment, but he said, "You're not out of the woods, because you're a compound heterozygote. You could cross over so we have to keep an eye on you.

My mom is homozygous for C282Y. My dad is a carrier. Everyone in my family—from me to my child to my mother and father—is affected in some way.

Genetic Testing

Genetic testing, which analyzes your DNA, confirms a diagnosis of hereditary hemochromatosis. It identifies the C282Y and H63D mutations and tells you if you are a heterozygote, homozygote, or compound heterozygote.

A doctor may order a liver biopsy for diagnostic purposes in at least three situations:

- *When available genetic tests are negative but iron tests are elevated (5–10 percent of cases of HH);*
- *When in homozygotes, compound heterozygotes, and rare heterozygotes, a liver biopsy may be necessary to determine the degree of iron overload in order to decide if phlebotomy is needed;*
- *When there is concern about possible cirrhosis.*

WHO SHOULD BE TESTED? Early detection is essential in preventing symptoms and organ damage. Therefore, if you, a relative or spouse has hemochromatosis, genetic testing acts as an early warning system for family members.

"Testing one individual provides information for the family," says Annette K. Taylor, M.S., Ph.D., President and Laboratory Director of Kimball Genetics in Denver, Colo. "Testing one person often starts a chain of events, and we end up testing several family members. Hemochromatosis is under-diagnosed. Sometimes it's not diagnosed until autopsy. The importance of DNA testing is to facilitate an early diagnosis and to identify family members at risk."

You should consider genetic testing and discuss testing with your physician if you have any of the following results or clinical features:

- *Elevated Transferrin Saturation*
    Women % saturation > 50%
    Men % saturation > 60%
- *Transferrin Saturation > 45% and Elevated Ferritin*
- *Your first degree relative had HH.*
- *Your first degree relative had a history of unknown liver disease, arthritis, diabetes mellitus, and you have high iron studies or abnormal liver tests.*

Genetic Counseling

Most people and families dealing with HH find that their physicians provide initial counseling and sufficient information. Many doctors, however, lack formal training in genetic diseases. Therefore, you may wish to talk to a specialist in genetic counseling.

WHAT IS GENETIC COUNSELING? "Genetic counseling is a communication process whereby the genetic counselor works with an individual or family either at risk for or already diagnosed with a genetic condition or trait," says Carol Walton, M.S., C.G.C., Director of the Graduate Program in Genetic Counseling at the University of Colorado Health Sciences Center. "The goals are to help the family understand their condition from the medical, scientific, and genetic aspects (Why do I have this? How did I get it? Did I inherit it? Is it new in me? Can I pass it on?) and to help facilitate decision-making. The family has to make complex decisions about medical management, genetic, and recurrence issues. The genetic counselor helps with the adjustment to the diagnosis from a social and psychological standpoint."

According to Walton, "The key aspect of genetic counseling is that it is a non-directive process. The genetic counselor does not give opinions. Rather, he or she helps the family recognize what their needs are and how the decisions they make are going to fit in with their family cultural and religious background. The counselor helps them come to the decision that they'll be most comfortable with, based on a good understanding of the information. Counselors also try to hook up people to external community resources, support groups, and family counseling resources."

FINDING AND SELECTING A GENETIC COUNSELOR. Both geneticists and genetic counselors provide genetic counseling. Geneticists are board-certified physicians specializing in genetic conditions. In addition, many physicians, usually working on a team with genetic counselors, also provide counseling.

If you are selecting a genetic counselor, it's wise to ask about credentials. Does the counselor have a degree in genetic counseling from an accredited master's level graduate program? Is he or she board certified by the American Board of Genetic Counseling (ABGC)? Some state legislatures, such as those in California and Utah, require licenses. Most academic medical centers have genetic counseling services. If you live in a rural area, ask if the centers provide outreach clinics.

RESOURCE: The National Society of Genetic Counselors, Inc. (NSGC) features a "ResourceLink" on its Web site that helps people locate genetic counseling services by state, city, and specialty. The NSGC is located at 233 Canterbury Dr., Wallingford, PA 19086. Phone: 610-872-7608; Web site: www.nsgc.org

RESOURCE: Check the list of HH support organizations in the Resources section at the end of this book. Many of them provide lists of expert physicians, geneticists, and genetic clinics.

INTERPRETING THE RESULTS OF GENETIC (DNA) TESTS. Now that you've had the genetic tests, what do the results mean? Here is a simple table to help you interpret the results:

AT RISK FOR HEREDITARY HEMOCHROMATOSIS AND IRON OVERLOAD	
C282Y/C282Y	Two abnormal genes, common mutation for HH
C282Y/H63D	Two abnormal genes, second most common mutation for HH

AT NO OR LOW RISK FOR HEREDITARY HEMOCHROMATOSIS	
H63D/H63D	Two abnormal genes, but not sufficient for HH
C282Y/Normal	One abnormal gene, common carrier
H63D/Normal	One abnormal gene, common carrier
Normal/Normal	Unaffected population *

There are cases of hereditary hemochromatosis not associated with mutations in the HFE gene.

In the following examples I will examine the six potential results of your DNA test report more carefully. Each discussion will begin with a depiction of your results as they may appear in the report (Note: In some reports C282Y is designated by Cys282Tyr and H63D by His63Asp).

RESULT #1:
- *C282Y: Homozygote for this mutation*
- *H63D: Normal genotype*

This result indicates that you have two copies (homozygote) of the major hemochromatosis mutation, C282Y. Approximately 1 in 100 persons of European descent have this genetic makeup. If your iron tests confirm iron overload, then hereditary hemochromatosis (HH) is likely. If your iron tests do not reveal iron overload, you are still at-risk during your lifetime to develop HH, and you need periodic monitoring.

The lifetime risk of elevated iron studies (transferrin saturation) from homozygous C282Y is 100 percent, and the lifetime risk of progressive iron overload in tissues is 58 percent. The risk of organ damage is proportional to the severity of iron overload; estimates range from 20 percent to 50 percent. Nonetheless, some homozygous patients fail to develop iron overload or organ damage. A liver biopsy is often required to confirm the degree of iron overload and the need for phlebotomy treatment. Your brothers and sisters are at risk for homozygous C282Y and development of HH, and both of your parents and all of your children will have at least one C282Y mutation.

RESULT #2:

- *C282Y: Heterozygote for this mutation*
- *H63D: Heterozygote for this mutation*

This result indicates that you have one copy of each (compound heterozygote) of two mutations associated with hemochromatosis, C282Y and H63D. The prevalence is approximately 2 to 3 per 100 persons of Northern European descent. If your iron tests confirm iron overload, then HH is likely. If iron tests do not confirm iron overload, you will need periodic monitoring. A liver biopsy is usually required to confirm the degree of iron overload and the need for phlebotomy treatment. The lifetime risk for iron overload is unknown but may approach 20 to 30 percent. Clinical signs, symptoms, or disease occur in as few as 1 to 2 percent of compound heterozygotes.

RESULT #3:

- *C282Y: Normal genotype*
- *H63D: Homozygote*

This result indicates that you have two copies of the H63D mutation, an event that occurs in approximately 1 in 28 persons in populations of European descent. Current studies indicate that this genetic makeup is not independently associated with HH. Some recommend iron studies to evaluate for iron overload, but in nearly all cases, the iron studies are normal.

RESULT #4:

- *C282Y: Heterozygote for this mutation*

◆ *H63D: Normal genotype*

This result indicates that you are a "carrier" of one C282Y mutation. This occurs in approximately 1 in 10 persons of Northern European extraction. Heterozygosity for C282Y may be associated with slight elevations in iron studies but does not independently cause HH. Iron studies are often recommended, but in most cases they are normal.

RESULT #5:
◆ *C282Y: Normal genotype*
◆ *H63D: Heterozygote*

This result indicates that you are a "carrier" of one H63D mutation. This occurs in approximately 1 in 4 persons of Northern European extraction. Heterozygosity for H63D is not associated with risk for HH.

RESULT #6:
◆ *C282Y: Normal genotype*
◆ *H63D: Normal genotype*

This result indicates a normal genetic makeup relative to HFE genes. You do not have either of the two known mutations associated with hemochromatosis, and the results rule out the most common genetic causes of hemochromatosis. However, some cases of HH (up to 10 percent) are due to other unidentified mutations. If you have iron overload, phlebotomy treatment may still be indicated.

CASE HISTORY. Genetic counselors create a family history chart to trace the genetic mutations of HH. (Figure 3, Pedigree of a Family with Hemochromatosis, is an example of one such chart.) Note that each one-half of a circle or square indicates the one gene inherited from each parent.

Reason for Request of Genetic Testing. The first detected case in this family was a male with high ferritin levels who was being treated by phlebotomy (➔). His father underwent genetic testing and was found to be homozygous for C282Y (see Figure 3-1). The father, who had remarried, wanted to find out whether the two children he had with his second wife had HH (see Figure 3-2). Testing indicated that his second wife

FIGURE 3: PEDIGREE OF A FAMILY WITH HEMOCHROMATOSIS

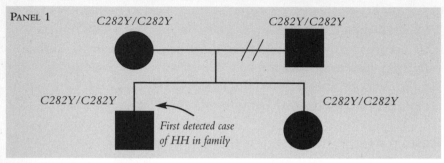

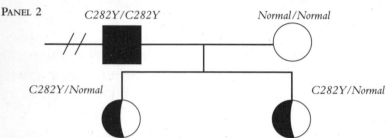

The father of the man who was first detected (Panel 1), divorced and remarried an unaffected woman (Normal/Normal). All their offspring are C28Y carriers (heterozygotes).

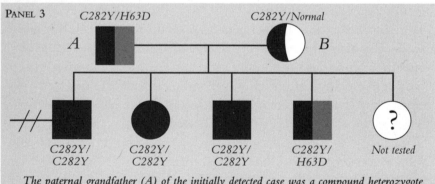

The paternal grandfather (A) of the initially detected case was a compound heterozygote and the paternal grandmother (B) was a C28Y carrier.

LEGEND 3: Details of this pedigree are discussed in the text. Men are shown as squares and women as circles. If the circle or square is completely filled, then the individual carries two mutations. If the circle or square is half filled, then the individual carries only one mutation. In each of the Panels, the father of the first detected case is indicated by the solid square to the right of the double diagonal crossing lines. Panel 1: The first detected case was a male with elevated iron and ferritin who was undergoing phlebotomy treatment (black arrow). Both of his parents were homozygous for the C282Y mutation of hemochromatosis. As a result, both he and his sister had hemochromatosis. Panel 2: His parents divorced and his father remarried an unaffected woman. Their two children were carriers of C282Y. Panel 3: Subsequent testing of aunts, uncles and grandparents yielded additional cases, of both C282Y homozygotes and compound heterozygotes, C282Y/H63D.

was negative for both C282Y and H63D and that his two daughters, therefore, were carriers. Interestingly, his ex-wife was tested and was homozygous for C282Y. Because both he and his ex-wife were both homozygous, both of his children by his first marriage were homozygous for C282Y.

Results of Additional Testing of the Family. At the top of Figure 3, we see that the grandfather was a compound heterozygote with one C282Y mutated gene and one H63D mutated gene. The grandmother was a carrier with one normal gene and one C282Y mutated gene (heterozygous for C282Y). The father, one aunt, and an uncle inherited both C282Y mutations (homozygous for C282Y). All of these three would be at risk for iron overload. Interestingly, the aunt had normal ferritin levels and is currently being monitored, but the uncle had iron overload and needed treatment. The sister had normal ferritin levels but the brother needed treatment. The other brother inherited one C282Y mutated gene and one H63D mutated gene (heterozygous for both), had high ferritin levels and was treated. Another aunt was not tested.

Outcomes: The father learned that his current wife had two normal genes, and his two daughters by this second marriage were carriers and not at risk for disease. The father felt relieved when he was given this information.

In addition, his daughters, HH-affected siblings, and ex-wife received potentially lifesaving information. This family is a good example of how the detection of a single case can lead to identification of the condition in relatives. Early detection through this type of case finding and follow-up can lead to treatment, prevent disease, and save lives.

Questions People Ask About Genetic Testing for Hemochromatosis

HOW FAR ALONG THE BRANCHES OF THE FAMILY TREE SHOULD WE TEST? As illustrated by the family pedigree shown in Figure 3, it is important to do genetic tests in first degree relatives of an affected individual, including brothers, sisters, mother, father, and offspring. Undiagnosed cases can be detected by this approach. However, there are several nuances to testing that deserve further discussion.

Let's suppose you have homozygous HH, two C282Y mutations. At a minimum, all of your offspring will be carriers of one gene of C282Y.

In this scenario, your spouse or partner should be tested. If this spouse or partner lacks any HFE mutation, then there would be no need for genetic testing of offspring. The genotype of all offspring would be heterozygous. If the partner were either homozygous for the C282Y or H63D HFE mutations, no additional testing of offspring would be needed because all would be affected and genotype C282Y/C282Y or C282Y/H63D. Testing of offspring is definitely indicated if the partner is a carrier of either C282Y or H63D as each child would be at risk for HH.

What is recommended if you are a carrier of C282Y (see Chapter 4)? You should inform your siblings and parents, and they should consider testing, at least for elevated iron saturation. Those with increased iron levels should undergo gene testing. Again, testing your spouse or reproductive partner is relevant. If your partner tests negative for HFE mutations, then no further gene testing of offspring is warranted. If the partner is either homozygous or heterozygous for HFE mutations, then gene testing of offspring is warranted. If your partner is homozygous, then there is a 50 percent chance that your offspring would be homozygous and develop HH. If the partner is heterozygous, then there is a 25 percent chance for HH (see Chapter 4 for more information).

The high prevalence of the HFE mutations in certain populations suggests that at least at some point in time, this mutation conferred some level of survival advantage. As suggested earlier, the C282Y mutation may reduce risk of iron deficiency in women and maintain higher rates of fertility. Perhaps this was a factor in the emergence of the high prevalence of the HFE mutation in the Celtic and Northern European populations.

HOW DO I TAKE A GENETIC TEST FOR HH? Genetic tests for HH should be considered in certain circumstances (see Who Should Be Tested?). If you fall in these categories, testing is relatively simple. In most cases, your doctor will send a sample of your blood to a laboratory.

Some labs also provide a kit that does the gene testing by using samples of cheek cells. The kit typically includes information about HH, directions for swabbing the inside surface of your cheek with sterile brushes, and directions for returning the sample for testing.

HOW MUCH DOES IT COST? Costs vary but generally range from $100+ to $400 per person. Ask if a discounted price is available for multiple tests of family members. In general, insurance companies will pay for the test.

HOW ACCURATE IS THE TEST? If you have the mutation, genetic testing for hemochromatosis is more than 99.9 percent accurate—and human or technical error accounts for the remaining .1 percent.

IF MY GENETIC TEST RESULTS DO NOT SHOW THAT I HAVE HH, DOES THAT MEAN I DON'T HAVE IRON OVERLOAD? No. Approximately 5 to 10 percent of people with a clinical diagnosis of hemochromatosis have negative DNA test results. Perhaps they have a genetic mutation that scientists have not yet discovered.

In any case, if your doctor has determined that you have iron overload, you need to be treated—no matter what the genetic tests reveal.

HOW REPUTABLE IS THE LAB? The Centers for Medicare and Medicaid Services (CMS) is the federal agency that regulates all laboratory testing, except research, performed on humans in the U.S. through the Clinical Laboratory Improvement Amendments (CLIA). To get and maintain a CLIA license, a lab must be inspected and then reinspected every two years.

The College of American Pathologists (CAP) has expertise in genetics, says Dr. Taylor, so CLIA allows CAP to inspect genetic labs (except in New York and Washington states, which have their own regulation and certification programs). CAP conducts a rigorous inspection program every two years that includes personal visits and proficiency testing. Not all genetic labs have CAP inspection so it's important to ask if the lab is CAP-certified.

RESOURCE: For a free voluntary listing of laboratories offering genetic testing and genetic clinics providing genetic evaluation and genetic counseling, as well as other information about medical genetics, access the publicly funded Web site, Gene Tests-Gene Clinics. Web site: www.genetests.org.

RESOURCE: For more information about CLIA, including a list of approved accrediting organizations, access the Centers for Medicare and Medicaid Services Web site. CMS, the federal agency responsible for administering CLIA, is located at 7500 Security Blvd., Baltimore, MD 21244-1850. Phone: 410-786-3000; Web site: www.cms.hhs.gov/clia

RESOURCE: The College of American Pathologists (CAP) is located at 325 Waukegan Rd., Northfield, IL 60093. Phone: 1-800-323-4040 (in Illinois, 847-832-7000); Web site: www.cap.org

HOW CONFIDENTIAL ARE THE RESULTS? By law, laboratories must report test results (including results of home collection kits) to the patient's health care professional. Not all labs will also send a copy of the results directly to you, so ask up front if that's an important consideration.

If you are concerned about confidentiality, you may want to make sure that you receive the results by mail, not by phone or fax. Of course, no lab should give out results of your tests to anyone other than your physician without a medical release from you, but it's a good idea to make sure of this by asking about the lab's routine procedures.

> RESOURCE: The Department of Health and Human Services recently issued a final regulation on medical records privacy requirements. For an explanation of the major provisions of the Health Insurance Portability and Accountability Act (HIPAA) privacy rule and how it affects laboratories, pathologists, and physicians, see "Special Report: HIPAA Privacy Rule Final Release," *Statline*, the College of American Pathologists newsletter, Aug. 14, 2002. Web site: www.cap.org

CAN GENETIC TEST RESULTS AFFECT MY LIFE OR HEALTH INSURANCE COVERAGE? CAN GENETIC TESTS RESULT IN JOB DISCRIMINATION? (See Chapter 8, Financial Impact of Hemochromatosis, for a discussion of genetic discrimination.)

In summary, this chapter explains several concepts about genes, genetic mutations, and the basis for hemochromatosis. Two genetic mutations, C282Y and H63D, account for more than 90 percent of the cases of HH. Asymptomatic carriers of both mutations are common and rarely, if ever, develop iron overload or HH.

We discussed several different combinations of results of genetic tests and presented examples to clarify the meaning of the results of these tests. In addition, current data indicates that some patients may have iron overload similar to HFE-associated hemochromatosis but lack mutations in the HFE gene on chromosome 6. Current genetic tests are accurate but may not define all cases of HH.

> *It is by presence of mind in untried emergencies*
> *that the native metal of a man is tested.*
> JAMES RUSSELL LOWELL
> *"Abraham Lincoln"*

4

THE CARRIER

What About Me?
What About My Family?

*My daughter was diagnosed with hemochromatosis. She told me to
get tested. My doctor said I was okay, that I wasn't even a carrier.*

*Then my daughter read the lab report and showed me where it said,
"The C282Y mutation was not detected. One copy of the H63D
mutation was identified (heterozygous for this mutation)."*

"Dad," she said, "that means you're a carrier."

GEORGE

I F SOMEONE IN YOUR FAMILY HAS JUST BEEN
diagnosed with hereditary hemochromatosis, you are probably
asking yourself, "What about me? Do I have HH or am I a carrier? Will my children have hemochromatosis?"

Obviously, if a close blood relative has HH, it's a warning sign that you
may need to be tested. Even if you don't have iron overload and HH, you
may be a carrier of one "silent," mutated hemochromatosis gene.

How does being a carrier affect your life? In this chapter, we will
explore the following topics:

- *What Is a Carrier?*
- *What Are My Chances of Being a Carrier or Having HH?*
    - ONE PARENT HAS HH DUE TO TWO MUTATIONS OF C282Y
    - ONE PARENT HAS HH DUE TO ONE MUTATION EACH OF C282Y AND H63D
    - RECOMMENDATIONS FOR GENE-TESTING WHEN A PARENT IS DIAGNOSED WITH HH
    - ONE PARENT IS A CARRIER OF ONE MUTATION OF C282Y
    - ONE PARENT IS A CARRIER OF ONE MUTATION OF H63D
    - RECOMMENDATIONS FOR GENE TESTING WHEN A PARENT IS A CARRIER
    - ONE SISTER OR BROTHER HAS HH DUE TO TWO MUTATIONS OF C282Y
    - ONE SISTER OR BROTHER HAS HH DUE TO ONE MUTATION EACH OF C282Y AND H63D
    - ONE SISTER OR BROTHER IS A CARRIER OF ONE MUTATION OF C282Y
    - ONE SISTER OR BROTHER IS A CARRIER OF ONE MUTATION OF H63D
  - A MORE DISTANT RELATION HAS HH OR IS A CARRIER
- *What Are the Chances of Passing Hemochromatosis to My Children?*
- *If I Am Only a Carrier, Can I Develop Iron Overload and Organ Damage?*
- *Should I Avoid Iron and Vitamin C Supplements? Alcohol?*
- *How Can I Find Out If I Am a Carrier?*

Note: I recommend that you read Chapter 3 for a background in the basic genetics of hemochromatosis before proceeding with this chapter. It is especially important to understand the two common genetic mutations for hemochromatosis, C282Y and H63D.

The genetics of hereditary hemochromatosis is incompletely defined at the time of this writing. Certainly it is clear that the majority of cases of HH in persons of European descent are related to the inheritance of two mutations of C282Y (majority) or one mutation each of C282Y and H63D (minority). Other mutations in the HFE gene, such as S65C, and mutations in other genes are under investigation.

A key point to remember is that HH refers to excessive iron accumulation in the body, but not all individuals with the above mutations have iron overload. It is better to consider the gene mutations in the following way. A person inherits the susceptibility to develop hemochromatosis via two common mutations, C282Y and H63D. However, the risk of HH is far greater for a person inheriting two mutations of C282Y compared to one mutation each of C282Y and H63D. A person who inherits two mutations of H63D is not at risk for HH.

In the text and tables of this chapter, I refer to the risk of hemochromatosis and iron overload primarily as it relates to the likelihood of inheriting either two mutations of C282Y or one mutation each of C282Y and H63D. The risk is further adjusted by the estimates for each of these inherited patterns to cause elevated iron studies (100 and 30 percent, respectively), and clinically apparent organ damage (20 and 2 percent, respectively).

What Is a Carrier?

A carrier is a person who is otherwise healthy but who has inherited one mutated gene for hemochromatosis from one parent. Carriers typically do not develop HH, iron overload, or clinical illness related to organ damage from iron.

> After my wife was diagnosed with hemochromatosis, we wrote all our relatives about HH. We got a letter back saying that my grandmother had iron overload …on my mother and father's side, six out of seven siblings died of heart attacks in their late thirties and forties. So I had the doctor check my ferritin. The test came back okay, and I thought I was home free.
>
> About a year or two later, my wife and I both had genetic testing. The test showed that my wife was double on the C282Y. I was a carrier of one bad gene, H63D. People tell me I'm lucky.
>
> PETE

In Chapter 3, I indicated that two genetic mutations, C282Y and H63D are relevant in terms of the risk of developing hemochromatosis. In the future, additional mutated genes may be discovered. For the following discussion and examples I focus only on C282Y and H63D mutations.

Given this information, you can see that there are potentially two types of carriers:

(1) a person carrying one C282Y mutation
(2) a person carrying one H63D mutation

Current studies suggest that approximately 10 percent of individuals of Northern European background carry the C282Y mutation and 25 percent carry the H63D mutation. Approximately 20 million Americans are carriers of C282Y, and 40 million are carriers of H63D.

Gene testing is not currently recommended for screening of national populations. Therefore, iron tests and gene tests usually detect those who are carriers or those with hemochromatosis, often after another member of the family has been diagnosed.

What Are My Chances of Being a Carrier or of Having HH?

Suppose you have recently been informed that one of your relatives—a parent, sibling, or more distant relation—has HH or is a carrier of one mutation of either C282Y or H63D. The following scenarios cover all the possibilities. In the first set of cases, the father is affected and the risk to you is then determined by your mother's genetic composition. Of course, if your mother is the affected parent, then your risk is determined by your father's genetic composition. In the second set of cases, I use a brother as the affected sibling, although, of course, the same results would occur with a sister. In addition, I also discuss the situation where the affected person is a distant relative.

One Parent Has HH Due to Two C282Y Mutations (TABLE 4A). Let's examine the situation in which your father has two mutations of C282Y. You and all your siblings will inherit one C282Y mutation from him. At a minimum, all of you would be carriers. But you also could be at risk for HH, depending upon your mother's genetic makeup. In this case, your mother should undergo genetic testing.

Case 1: Mother lacks either the C282Y or H63D mutation. Remember, you inherit one gene from your father and one from your mother. In this case, you and your brothers and sisters inherit one C282Y mutation from your father and no mutation from your mother. You and all of your siblings are carriers of one mutation of C282Y.

Case 2: Mother is a carrier of one mutation of C282Y. You and each of your siblings receive one C282Y gene from your father, but you also have a 1 in 2 chance (50 percent chance) of receiving the mutated C282Y gene from your mother. If this occurs, you are at risk for iron overload (lifetime risk approaches 100 percent) and would need monitoring, follow-up, and probably phlebotomy treatment. If you receive the normal gene from your mother, then you are a carrier. In other words, half of the offspring born from your mother and father are at risk for HH and half would be carriers of the C282Y mutation.

Case 3: Mother is a carrier of one mutation of H63D. Once again, you and each of your siblings receive one C282Y gene from your father. But in this case, you also have a 50 percent chance of receiving the mutated H63D gene from your mother. If this occurs, you have one C282Y mutation and one H63D mutation and might develop iron overload and HH (approximate lifetime risk of 30 percent). You will likely need additional monitoring, liver biopsy, and possibly phlebotomy treatment.

If you receive the normal gene from your mother, then you are a carrier, possessing only one mutation of C282Y. In other words, half of the offspring borne from your mother and father have one mutation each of C282Y and H63D and are at risk for iron overload and HH. The other half are carriers of one C282Y mutation.

TABLE 4A: RISK OF HH AND CARRIER STATE IN OFFSPRING WHEN ONE PARENT HAS HH DUE TO TWO C282Y MUTATIONS

GENE TESTING RESULTS OF NAIVE (OTHER) PARENT

		ONE MUTATION OF	
	NORMAL	C282Y	H63D
THE RISK IN OFFSPRING FOR:			
C282Y CARRIER	100%	50%	50%
HH, C282Y/C282Y	0%	50%★	0%★
HH, C282Y/H63D	0%	0%★	50%★
IRON OVERLOAD★	0%	50%	15%
ORGAN DAMAGE★	0%	10%	1%

*Indicates groups at risk for development of iron overload, HH, and organ damage related to iron accu-
mulation. Lifetime risk of iron overload is calculated by multiplying the risk of HH mutations in offspring by 1 for HH, C282Y/C282Y mutations, and 0.3 for HH, C282Y/H63D mutations. Risk
for clinically-apparent, organ damage is calculated by multiplying risk of HH mutation by .2 for HH,
C282Y/C282Y, and .02 for HH, C282Y/H63D.

ONE PARENT HAS HH DUE TO ONE MUTATION EACH OF C282Y AND H63D (TABLE 4B).

Individuals who inherit one each of the C282Y and H63D mutations may also develop iron overload and HH. Suppose your father has HH due to one mutation each of C282Y and H63D. You and all your siblings have a 50 percent chance of inheriting either one C282Y mutation or one H63D mutation from him. At a minimum, all of you would be carriers of one of these two mutations. But you may also be at risk for HH, depending upon your mother's genetic makeup. Your mother should undergo genetic testing.

Case 1: Mother lacks either the C282Y or H63D mutation. Remember, you will inherit one gene from your father and one from your mother. In this case you and your brothers and sisters have a 50 percent chance of inheriting either one C282Y mutation or one H63D mutation from your father and no mutation from your mother. Half the offspring are carriers of a single C282Y mutation and half are carriers of a single H63D mutation. None will develop HH.

Case 2: Mother is a carrier of one mutation of C282Y. You and each of your siblings inherit either one C282Y mutation or one H63D mutation from your father. Each of you has a 50 percent chance of inheriting another C282Y mutation from your mother. In this situation, 25 percent of the offspring are carriers of C282Y; 25 percent are carriers of H63D; 25 percent have one mutation each and are at risk for HH; and 25 percent have two C282Y mutations and HH.

Case 3: Mother is a carrier of one mutation of H63D. You and each of your siblings inherit either one C282Y mutation or one H63D mutation from your father. Each of you has a 50 percent chance of inheriting another H63D mutation from your mother. In this situation,

25 percent of the offspring are carriers of C282Y; 25 percent are carriers of H63D; 25 percent have one mutation each and are at risk for HH; and 25 percent have two H63D mutations. Individuals with two H63D mutations do not develop HH.

TABLE 4B: RISK OF HH AND CARRIER STATE IN OFFSPRING WHEN ONE PARENT HAS HH DUE TO ONE C282Y MUTATION AND ONE H63D MUTATION

| | GENE TESTING RESULTS OF NAIVE (OTHER) PARENT | | |
| | ONE MUTATION OF | | |
	NORMAL	C282Y	H63D
THE RISK IN OFFSPRING FOR:			
C282Y CARRIER	50%	25%	25%
H63D CARRIER	50%	25%	25%
HH, C282Y/C282Y	0%	25%★	0%★
HH, C282Y/H63D	0%	25%★	25%★
H63D/H63D (NOT HH)	0%	0%	25%
IRON OVERLOAD★	0%	33%	8%
ORGAN DAMAGE★	0%	5.5%	0.5%

Indicates groups at risk for development of iron overload, HH, and organ damage related to iron accumulation. Lifetime risk of iron overload is calculated by multiplying the risk of HH mutations in offspring by 1 for HH, C282Y/C282Y mutations, and 0.3 for HH, C282Y/H63D mutations. Risk for clinically apparent organ damage is calculated by multiplying risk of HH mutation by .2 for HH, C282Y/C282Y, and .02 for HH, C282Y/H63D.

RECOMMENDATIONS FOR GENE-TESTING WHEN A PARENT IS DIAGNOSED WITH HH. The above discussion provides a rationale for genetic testing in the circumstance where one parent is known to have HH. The first step is to perform gene testing of the other (naive) parent to define the risk of transmission to children. If the gene tests in this parent are normal (negative), then all offspring are carriers, each inheriting only one mutation from the father. Because the carrier state is not associated with risk for HH, no further testing or liver biopsy is warranted.

In the case where the father has HH due to two C282Y mutations, all offspring would be carriers of one mutation of C282Y. In the case where the father has HH due to one mutation each of C282Y and H63D, half the offspring would carry one mutation of C282Y and half would carry one mutation of H63D. Further genetic testing of these offspring is not necessary since there is no risk for HH. Some have advo-cated iron studies, however, because there may be additional HFE muta-tions not detected by current genetic tests. Offspring with high iron studies may need liver biopsy.

Genetic testing should be performed in offspring when the naive parent's gene tests are positive for C282Y or H63D, or the naive parent is unavailable for gene testing. In these circumstances the risk for HH in a given person cannot be defined, and iron testing may not be suffi-ciently accurate, especially in younger individuals. Genetic testing will define the risk for HH and the need for additional studies, including a liver biopsy. Offspring who test positive for either two mutations of C282Y or one mutation each of C282Y and H63D need iron studies, liver biopsy, treatment, and long-term follow-up.

ONE PARENT IS A CARRIER OF ONE MUTATION OF C282Y (TABLE 4C). Suppose your father has one mutation of C282Y. You and all your siblings have a 50 percent chance of inheriting the C282Y mutation from him. At a minimum, 50 percent of you and your siblings are carriers. But you may also be at risk for HH, depending upon your mother's genetic makeup. In this case your mother should undergo genetic testing.

Case 1: Mother lacks either the C282Y or H63D mutation. Remember, you inherit one gene from your father and one from your mother. In this scenario, you and your brothers and sisters would have a 50 percent chance of inheriting one C282Y mutation from your father and no other mutation from your mother. Half the offspring would be carriers of one mutation of C282Y.

Case 2: Mother is a carrier of one mutation of C282Y. You and each of your siblings have a 50 percent chance of inheriting one C282Y mutation from your father, but you also have a 50 percent chance of inheriting a C282Y mutation from your mother. The likeli-hood of inheriting both C282Y mutations and developing HH is 1 in 4, or a 25 percent chance. The likelihood of being a carrier of one muta-tion is 2 in 4, or a 50 percent chance, and the likelihood of being unaf-fected is 1 in 4, or a 25 percent chance.

Case 3: Mother is a Carrier of one mutation of H63D. You and each of your siblings have a 50 percent chance of inheriting one C282Y gene from your father and also a 50 percent chance of inheriting the

H63D mutation from your mother. There is a 25 percent chance that you would inherit both mutations and be at risk for HH and iron overload. The likelihood of being a carrier of C282Y is 1 in 4 (25 percent chance); the likelihood of being a carrier of H63D is 1 in 4 (25 percent chance); and the likelihood of being unaffected is 1 in 4 (25 percent chance).

TABLE 4C: RISK OF HH AND CARRIER STATE IN OFFSPRING WHEN ONE PARENT IS A CARRIER OF ONE C282Y MUTATION

GENE TESTING RESULTS OF NAIVE (OTHER) PARENT

ONE MUTATION OF

THE RISK IN OFFSPRING FOR:	NORMAL	C282Y	H63D
C282Y CARRIER	50%	50%	25%
H63D CARRIER	0%	0%	25%
HH, C282Y/C282Y	0%	25%★	0%★
HH, C282Y/H63D	0%	0%★	25%★
H63D/H63D (NOT HH)	0%	0%	0%
IRON OVERLOAD★	0%	25%	8%
ORGAN DAMAGE★	0%	5%	0.5%

Indicates groups at risk for development of iron overload, HH, and organ damage related to iron accumulation. Lifetime risk of iron overload is calculated by multiplying the risk of HH mutations in offspring by 1 for HH, C282Y/C282Y mutations, and 0.3 for HH, C282Y/H63D mutations. Risk for clinically apparent organ damage is calculated by multiplying risk of HH mutation by .2 for HH, C282Y/C282Y, and .02 for HH, C282Y/H63D.

ONE PARENT IS A CARRIER OF ONE MUTATION OF H63D (TABLE 4D).

Suppose your father has one mutation of H63D. You and all your siblings have a 50 percent chance of inheriting the H63D mutation from him. At a minimum, 50 percent of you and your siblings are carriers, but you may also be at risk for HH, depending upon your mother's genetic makeup. In this case your mother should undergo genetic testing.

Case 1: Mother lacks either the C282Y or H63D mutation. Remember, you will inherit one gene from your father and one from your mother. In this scenario you and your brothers and sisters would have a 50 percent chance of inheriting one H63D mutation from your father and no other mutation from your mother. Half the offspring would be carriers of one mutation of H63D.

Case 2: Mother is a carrier of one mutation of C282Y. You and each of your siblings have a 50 percent chance of inheriting one

H63D mutation from your father, but you also have a 50 percent chance of inheriting a C282Y mutation from your mother. The likelihood of inheriting both mutations and developing HH is 1 in 4, or a 25 percent chance. The likelihood of being a carrier of either the C282Y or H63D mutation is 2 in 4, or a 50 percent chance, and the likelihood of being unaffected is 1 in 4, or a 25 percent chance.

Case 3: Mother is a carrier of one mutation of H63D. You and each of your siblings have a 50 percent chance of inheriting one H63D gene from your father and also a 50 percent chance of inheriting another H63D mutation from your mother. There is a 1 in 4 or 25 percent chance that you would inherit both mutations, but you would not develop either HH or iron overload. The likelihood of being a carrier of H63D is 2 in 4, or a 50 percent chance, and the likelihood of being unaffected is 1 in 4, or a 25 percent chance.

TABLE 4D: RISK OF HH AND CARRIER STATE IN OFFSPRING WHEN ONE PARENT IS A CARRIER OF ONE H63D MUTATION

GENE TESTING RESULTS OF NAIVE (OTHER) PARENT

	NORMAL	ONE MUTATION OF C282Y	H63D
THE RISK IN OFFSPRING TO BE:			
C282Y CARRIER	0%	25%	0%
H63D CARRIER	50%	25%	50%
HH, C282Y/C282Y	0%	0%★	0%★
HH, C282Y/H63D	0%	25%★	0%★
H63D/H63D (NOT HH)	0%	0%	25%
IRON OVERLOAD★	0%	8%	0%
ORGAN DAMAGE★	0%	0.5%	0%

Indicates groups at risk for development of iron overload, HH, and organ damage related to iron accumulation. Lifetime risk of iron overload is calculated by multiplying the risk of HH mutations in offspring by 1 for HH, C282Y/C282Y mutations, and 0.3 for HH, C282Y/H63D mutations. Risk for clinically apparent organ damage is calculated by multiplying risk of HH mutation by .2 for HH, C282Y/C282Y, and .02 for HH, C282Y/H63D.

RECOMMENDATIONS FOR GENE TESTING WHEN A PARENT IS A CARRIER. When one parent is known to be a carrier of either C282Y or H63D, the first step is to perform gene testing of the naive parent to define the risk of transmission to the offspring. If the gene tests in the naive parent are normal (negative), then only 50 percent of the offspring are carriers, each inheriting only one mutation from the father. The others are unaffected.

Because the carrier state is not associated with risk for HH, no further testing or a liver biopsy of the offspring is warranted. Some have advocated iron studies, however, because there may be additional HFE mutations not detected by current genetic tests. Offspring with high iron studies may need further evaluation.

Genetic testing should be performed in offspring when one parent is positive for C282Y and the other is positive for either C282Y or H63D; one parent is positive for H63D and the other is positive for C282Y; or the second parent is unavailable for gene testing. In these circumstances the risk for HH in a given person cannot be defined, and iron testing may not be sufficiently accurate, especially in younger individuals. Genetic testing will define the risk for HH and the need for additional studies, including a liver biopsy. Offspring who test positive for either two mutations of C282Y or one mutation each of C282Y and H63D need iron studies and follow up which could include liver biopsy and treatment.

ONE SISTER OR BROTHER HAS HH DUE TO TWO MUTATIONS OF C282Y.

In this circumstance, your sibling must have inherited one C282Y mutation from your father and one from your mother. Although you too are at risk for HH, the magnitude of your risk cannot be precisely defined without knowing the results of your parents' genetic tests. If you know the genetic test results of your parents, then you can determine your risk of being a carrier, C282Y/C282Y, C282Y/H63D, or having iron overload and organ damage from Tables 4A through 4D.

In the absence of genetic testing of the parents, one can only infer the various potential possibilities of C282Y and H63D in the parents and give a range of risk. The following is an example of a range of risk determination for susceptibility of genes for HH or iron overload when one of your siblings has HH due to two mutations of C282Y:

		RISK FOR OFFSPRING	
		INHERITED HH TENDENCY	LIFETIME RISK OF IRON OVERLOAD
POSSIBLE COMBINATIONS IN PARENTS			
C282Y/C282Y	C282Y/C282Y	100%	100%
C282Y/C282Y	C282Y/NONE	50%	50%
C282Y/NONE	C282Y/NONE	25%	25%
C282Y/H63D	C282Y/NONE	50%	33%
C282Y/H63D	C282Y/H63D	75%	40%

This analysis indicates that you have a 25 to 100 percent chance of having iron overload in your lifetime when one of your siblings has HH due to two C282Y mutations. Obviously, this range of risk is high, and you should undergo both iron and gene testing.

ONE SISTER OR BROTHER HAS HH DUE TO ONE MUTATION EACH OF C282Y AND H63D. Your sibling must have received the C282Y mutation from one parent and the H63D mutation from your other parent. Once again, your risk cannot be determined precisely unless genetic tests are available for both parents.

Here is the analysis for determining your range of risk of developing HH in this circumstance:

		RISK FOR OFFSPRING	
		INHERITED HH TENDENCY	LIFETIME RISK OF IRON OVERLOAD
POSSIBLE COMBINATIONS IN PARENTS			
H63D/NONE	C282Y/NONE	25%	8%
H63D/H63D	C282Y/NONE	50%	15%
H63D/C282Y	C282Y/NONE	50%	33%
H63D/NONE	C282Y/C282Y	50%	15%
H63D/H63D	C282Y/C282Y	100%	30%
H63D/C282Y	C282Y/C282Y	100%	65%
H63D/NONE	C282Y/H63D	25%	8%
H63D/H63D	C282Y/H63D	50%	15%
H63D/C282Y	C282Y/H63D	75%	40%

This analysis indicates that you have an 8 to 65 percent chance of having iron overload in your lifetime when one of your siblings has HH due to one mutation each of C282Y and H63D. Obviously, this range of risk is also high, and you should undergo both iron and gene testing.

ONE SISTER OR BROTHER IS A CARRIER OF ONE MUTATION OF C282Y. In this circumstance, your sibling must have received one C282Y mutation from either your father or your mother. The carrier status of your sibling implies that at least one of your parents would have to be a carrier. Although you are at risk for HH, the magnitude of your risk cannot be precisely defined without the knowledge derived from genetic testing of your parents. If the results of genetic testing of your parents are known, then you can determine your risk of carrier, C282Y/C282Y, C282Y/H63D, or HH and iron overload from Tables 4A through 4D.

In the absence of genetic testing of the parents, one can only infer the various potential possibilities of C282Y and H63D in the parents and give a range of risk. Although you are at risk for HH, the magnitude of your risk is much lower than the risk if your sibling has HH. If one parent has HH and the other is a carrier, your risk of HH is 50 percent. If both are carriers, your risk is 25 percent, and if only one were a carrier, then your risk is 0 percent.

		RISK FOR OFFSPRING	
		INHERITED HH TENDENCY	LIFETIME RISK OF IRON OVERLOAD
POSSIBLE COMBINATIONS IN PARENTS			
C282Y/None	None/None	0%	0%
C282Y/None	C282Y/None	25%	25%
C282Y/None	C282Y/H63D	50%	33%
C282Y/None	C282Y/C282Y	50%	50%
H63D/None	C282Y/None	25%	8%
H63D/None	C282Y/H63D	25%	8%
H63D/None	C282Y/C282Y	50%	15%

In other words, in the absence of genetic testing of your parents, when your sibling is a carrier of one mutation of C282Y, you have a 0 to 50 percent chance of having iron overload. If there is no family history of HH, iron overload or suspicious clinical events, such as unexplained cirrhosis, then your risk of HH is very low, close to 0 percent. Why? Because it is at least 20 times more likely that only one of your parents is a carrier of C282Y, compared to any of the other possible combinations noted above. So when one of your siblings is a carrier, you should undergo iron testing but have gene testing only if the iron tests are abnormal.

ONE SISTER OR BROTHER IS A CARRIER OF ONE MUTATION OF H63D. The considerations in this circumstance are very similar to those encountered for the situation where your sibling is a carrier of one mutation of C282Y. If genetic tests of parents are known, then you can determine your risk by examining Tables 4A through 4D.

However, if gene tests of parents are not available, your risk for HH can only be inferred. If there is no family history of HH or clinical events suspicious for HH, then your risk of HH is very low. The most likely possibility is that either one or both of your parents are carriers of one mutation of H63D. Because this is 50 times more likely than any possible combination that could lead to HH, your lifetime risk of developing HH is close to 0 percent. For these reasons you should only have gene testing if iron studies are abnormal.

A MORE DISTANT RELATION HAS HH OR IS A CARRIER. The above discussion concerning your risk of HH is pertinent only when the initially diagnosed case is a close or first-degree relative. Occasionally, individuals learn of a cousin, aunt, uncle, or grandparent that may have had HH. Current recommendations suggest that you undergo iron testing, with genetic testing reserved for those family members with elevated iron studies.

What Are the Chances of Passing Hemochromatosis To My Children?

The risk that your offspring will develop hemochromatosis is dependent upon the results of genetic testing of your spouse or parental partner. Tables 4C and 4D define the risk of HH based upon genetic tests in partners of carriers.

I recommend genetic testing of the spouse or parental partner to determine the risk in the offspring. There is an approximately 10 percent chance that the partner is a carrier of C282Y mutation and a 25 percent chance that the partner is a carrier of H63D. The risk of HH in your children is 0 percent if your partner lacks C282Y and H63D mutations.

If I Am Only a Carrier, Can I Develop Iron Overload and Organ Damage?

This is a very common question. The medical literature, prior to the availability of genetic testing, suggested that "carriers," based on iron studies, might be at risk for disease of the heart, joints, coagulation system, type II diabetes mellitus, and liver. However, many of these carriers may actually have had HH or secondary hemochromatosis.

Recent studies using genetic tests indicate that carriers are essentially healthy. There is little to no evidence that carriers develop organ damage, clinical problems related to iron overload, liver disease, or premature death.

A few recent findings are noteworthy. Patients with HH have an increased risk of cardiac complications, but the risk in carriers is unclear. Three population-based studies suggest that the risk of coronary artery disease, myocardial infarction, and death from cardiovascular disease is increased in carriers. Rasmussen measured HFE mutations in 243 patients with coronary disease and 535 matched controls and found that coronary disease was 2.7 times more likely in carriers of the C282Y mutation. A Finnish group followed 1150 men over many years and found a 2.3-fold increase in the rate of myocardial infarction among 77 participants who were carriers of C282Y. Another study from the Netherlands examined cardiovascular death in 12,239 women and observed that C282Y carriers had 1.5-fold higher death rate for myocardial infarction, 2.4-fold higher death rate due to cerebrovascular disease, and 1.6-fold higher death rate for total cardiovascular disease.

Although, the above data suggest an association of C282Y carrier state and risk of cardiovascular disease, other studies refute these findings. A U.S. study of 30,916 white adults, aged 25 to 98, assessed the prevalence of coronary artery disease, risk factors for atherosclerosis, and frequency of HFE mutations. HFE carriers had a prevalence of coronary disease and atherosclerosis equivalent to unaffected individuals. A recent large angiographic study from Italy failed to demonstrate any relationship between the HFE carrier state and the risk of either coronary artery disease or myocardial infarction. Others have failed to confirm an association between the HFE carrier state and the risk of coronary disease, myocardial infarction, and cardiovascular death. At the time of this writing, any association of carrier state with cardiovascular disease is questionable.

Another prominent cardiac manifestation of HH is cardiomyopathy (weakening of the heart muscle), particularly with the blockade of the conduction system of the heart, and cardiac failure. The relationship, if any, of the carrier state of HFE mutations to cardiomyopathy is unclear, as two recent studies have given somewhat contradictory results. In both studies, the prevalence of the C282Y mutation was similar between patients with cardiomyopathy and the controls, indicating no relationship. In contrast, one study observed a 1.6-fold increase in H63D mutation in those with cardiomyopathy. Because H63D is not associated with a significant increase in iron, the investigators suggested that H63D may simply be a marker for another, as yet unidentified, gene relevant to cardiomyopathy. Nonetheless, there is little evidence that carriers of HFE mutations are at risk for cardiomyopathy.

Although arthritis and calcification of joint cartilage is a feature of HH, carriers are spared this complication. One hundred twenty-eight patients from the United Kingdom, with a pattern of joint symptoms and damage consistent with joint injury from HH, underwent testing for HFE mutations. The prevalence of HH was higher in the patients than in the general population, confirming the known relationship between HH and joint disease. However, the prevalence of C282Y and H63D carriers was similar to that of the general population, indicating no relationship of the carrier state to joint disease.

Some studies have suggested that carriers of HFE mutations may also have an increased frequency of mutations in a specific clotting factor, called factor V Leiden. The latter mutation would increase the risk for the clotting of veins in the body. Two recent reports, one from the United Kingdom and the other from Wales, indicate that carriers of HFE mutations are not at risk for either mutations in the clotting factor or for formation of venous clots.

Untreated HH is clearly associated with the development of Type II diabetes mellitus in late adult life. In contrast, recent studies of the prevalence of C282Y or H63D mutations in Type II diabetes have given conflicting results. Sampson and colleagues examined the prevalence of HFE mutations in 220 men with known Type II diabetes and compared results to non-diabetic controls. The prevalence of C282Y and H63D was similar in the two groups, failing to demonstrate any relationship of HFE mutations to diabetes. Another study compared clinical expression and sensitivity to insulin between diabetics with HFE mutations and diabetics without HFE mutations. This study failed to demonstrate an effect of HFE mutations on either the severity of diabetes or the response to insulin.

Other studies have demonstrated opposite results. These suggest that carriers of C282Y are at increased risk of diabetes, that the response to insulin is blunted, and that carriers of H63D may be prone to diabetic kidney disease. At the time of this writing, any association of the carrier state with Type II diabetes mellitus is questionable.

Serum iron tests and liver iron concentration may be increased in carriers of HFE mutations. However, there is little evidence that carriers are either at risk for liver disease from iron overload or that HFE mutations worsen severity or rates of progression of other liver diseases. When iron overload occurs, it is typically due to co-morbid disease, such as alcoholism, viral hepatitis, or chronic transfusion therapy.

One recent study found no increase in fibrosis or the severity of liver disease due to HFE mutations between groups of patients with various liver diseases. Another study showed that the proportion of patients who were carriers of C282Y was no different between patients on a liver transplant waiting list and the general population. Others have failed to confirm an association of carrier state with either worsening of alcoholic liver disease, nonalcoholic fatty liver, liver cancer, or hepatitis C. The general consensus is that carriers of HFE mutations are generally healthy, not at-risk for iron overload, have essentially normal liver function, and do not require extensive evaluation, follow-up, or treatment.

Should I Avoid Iron and Vitamin C Supplements? Alcohol?

Here's the backdrop: Twenty years ago, I got a call from an older cousin who said he had hemochromatosis. He told me to check my iron levels. My doctor said I didn't have HH, and that was the end of that.

Another backdrop: I had high liver enzymes in my twenties, but the doctor said to ignore it. Years later, I got very, very tired—so tired that I could hardly get from the sofa to a chair. My liver enzymes were high. My ferritin levels were high. When I told the doctor about my cousin, he said it was most probably HH and did a liver biopsy. That's how I found out I had hepatitis C.

My iron levels went high on interferon treatment for the hepatitis, and my doctor told me to get a genetic test. The test showed I have a defective gene. It took a couple of phlebotomies to get the ferritin level down, but after treatment was over, I never had trouble again.

I'm a carrier. I explained the whole situation to my sons and told them the odds were slim that they would have it.

Meanwhile, my cousin with HH is now 68—and he's as healthy as a horse!

DANNY

Rare cases of iron overload have occurred in patients who are carriers of the C282Y mutation. In general, these patients have had additional co-morbidities (such as alcoholism, viral hepatitis, excessive iron intake, or chronic transfusions) that would favor iron accumulation. For these reasons, it is common to recommend avoidance of iron-containing supplements or multivitamins and to limit alcohol use to 2 ounces or less per week. Vitamin C may enhance intestinal iron absorption and should be avoided.

How Can I Find Out If I Am A Carrier?

You can find out if you are a carrier by taking a gene test. (See Chapter 3, Gene Testing, for more information about testing, selecting a lab, and genetic counseling.)

Ice and iron cannot be welded.

ROBERT LOUIS STEVENSON

5

HOW HEMOCHROMATOSIS DAMAGES YOUR BODY

Effects of Iron Overload on the Liver, Heart, Pancreas, Joints, & Endocrine System

I started getting bronze patches on my jaw and temple, like shadows or dirt. I rubbed, but they didn't come off.

The patches get lighter with phlebotomies and darker when the iron builds up. Two little streaks on each side of my face are darker than the rest of my skin, a rusty color.

I'm like the Tin Man in The Wizard of Oz—*but I'd rather be Dorothy.*

NATALIE

WHEN DOCTORS DIAGNOSE YOU WITH HEMO-chromatosis, they prescribe phlebotomy treatments to get rid of the iron buildup and to prevent damage to your body's organs. If you are lucky enough to be diagnosed and treated early, you can expect to live a normal lifespan.

Unfortunately, your diagnosis may have been delayed. A CDC-supported survey, published in 1999, found that 67 percent of people with symptoms were first told they had a specific condition, such as diabetes, rather than the underlying cause—hemochromatosis. Furthermore, people reported that they had symptoms for an average of 10 years and went to an average of 3.5 physicians before they were diagnosed with HH.

Without prompt and proper treatment, iron buildup can cause liver and heart disease, diabetes, impotence, loss of menstrual periods, infertility, hair loss, bronze-colored skin, and other conditions. If the damage has already occurred, treatment may stop the disease from progressing, but may not be able to reverse the damage.

In addition to treating the underlying hemochromatosis with regular phlebotomy, you should consult appropriate medical specialists if you have clinical signs of disease. In this chapter, I describe the damage that can occur to organs as excess iron accumulates in your body:

- *Overview*
- *Iron Accumulation Over Time: Phases of Hemochromatosis*
- *Signs and Symptoms of Hemochromatosis*
- *Signs and Symptoms Due to Liver Disease*
    - CIRRHOSIS
        - Jaundice and Other Signs
        - Ascites and Edema
        - Varices
        - Encephalopathy
        - Impairment of Synthetic and Metabolic Functions
- *Signs and Symptoms Due to the Involvement of Other Organs*
    - HEART
    - PANCREAS
    - ENDOCRINE SYSTEM
    - SKIN
    - BONES AND JOINTS
    - INFECTION
- *Summary*

Overview

When hemochromatosis patients come to me for evaluation of their symptoms and clinical problems, I subdivide their symptoms into two categories. The first category includes symptoms due to the damage of organs known to be affected by HH and iron overload. The second category includes symptoms that may be due to other diseases or conditions. For example, thyroid disease is common in the general population, and it is not unusual for someone with hemochromatosis to also have thyroid disease. The two may be coincidental but not connected. In the following chapter, we focus on organ damage clearly linked to iron overload.

Iron Accumulation Over Time: Phases of Hemochromatosis

What is the progression of iron overload over time? In hereditary hemochromatosis, a rough relationship exists among the following three factors: age, level of iron accumulation, and clinical signs of organ damage.

AGE	TOTAL BODY IRON ACCULUMATION	CLINICAL SIGNS AND SYMPTOMS
0–20 YRS	0–10 G	NONE
20–40 YRS	10–20 G	IRON OVERLOAD
>40 YRS	>20 G	ORGAN DAMAGE

Iron begins to accumulate in early childhood, although the level of accumulation usually remains modest until adult life. Iron buildup of up to 5 grams is considered clinically insignificant and does not seem to affect health or produce symptoms. During this asymptomatic period, the range of iron tests may be quite broad, ranging from normal to very high and overlaying with symptomatic patients (Table 5A).

TABLE 5A. IRON STUDIES IN PATIENTS WITH HH

	NORMAL SUBJECTS	ASYMPTOMATIC	SYMPTOMATIC
SERUM IRON (UG/DL)	60–180	150–280	180–300
TRANSFERRIN SATURATION (%)	20–45	45–100	80–100
FERRITIN (NG/ML)			
MEN	20–200	150–1000	500–6000
WOMEN	15–150	120–1000	500–6000
HEPATIC IRON (UG/G)	300–1500	2000–10,000	8000–30,000
HEPATIC IRON INDEX	<1.0	1.0 TO >1.9	>1.9
LIVER IRON STAIN	0 TO 1+	2+ TO 4+	3+ TO 4+

As iron continues to accumulate, iron tests become abnormal, but organ function is still preserved. Organ damage typically doesn't show up until people age (over 40) and have more than 10 grams of iron stored in their tissues and organs.

Currently, many patients are diagnosed during a routine physical examination or a screening (of family members of an affected individual or of the general population). More than 75 percent of newly discovered cases have no symptoms, and much less than 25 percent have cirrhosis, diabetes, or skin pigmentation. If you start phlebotomy treatments prior to advanced age, the development of cirrhosis or diabetes mellitus, or the accumulation of less than 10 grams of iron, you can prevent clinical consequences and death related to hemochromatosis.

Patients with identical genetic tests (for example, two individuals who are both homozygous for C282Y) may have different rates of iron accumulation and risk of organ damage. The hepatic iron index (HII) represents the amount of iron in liver biopsies and adjusts for the age- and gender-related differences. The range of the HII in homozygous hemochromatosis is large. Some people will have an HII of 2, others of 10; 15 percent have an HII less than 1.9. Thus, the rate of iron accumulation varies considerably among HH patients.

Signs and Symptoms of Hemochromatosis

As I've stated, you might not have any symptoms in the early stages of HH. Later, usually after the third or fourth decade of life, substantial iron accumulates and symptoms emerge. Two phases characterize the symptomatic stage of hemochromatosis: an early phase with nonspecific complaints, such as fatigue, and a later phase with symptoms related to organ dysfunction.

> *I hit my 40s and never knew you start getting lethargic at 40! I'm used to going all day long, and now I can't function without a daily nap.*
>
> DON

In addition to fatigue, other symptoms in the early phase include lack of energy, lethargy, weakness, apathy, weight loss, aching of muscles and joints, impotence, abnormal liver tests, or nonspecific abdominal discomforts. None of these symptoms is unique, specific, or diagnostic of hemochromatosis.

However, a doctor's examination may reveal an enlarged liver, abnormal liver tests, skin pigmentation, diabetes, and heart enlargement. These symptoms of the later phase of HH are unique to specific organ dysfunction (see below) and appear as excessive iron progressively damages the cells and tissue of the organ.

Signs and Symptoms Due to Liver Disease

Because the liver is one of the main organs that regulates iron metabolism, many people with hemochromatosis find they have liver damage from iron overload. Without phlebotomy treatment, it is estimated that up to 50 percent of men and 25 percent of women with HH will develop clinically evident complications.

Approximately 50 to 75 percent of HH-related deaths are due to either complications of cirrhosis or hepatoma (liver cancer). A recent Danish study examined causes of death in 179 patients and found that hepatic failure due to cirrhosis was the cause in 32 percent, and cirrhosis with liver cancer was the cause in 23 percent. This study also demonstrated that survival of HH was higher in those without cirrhosis or diabetes and that phlebotomy, even in cirrhotics or diabetics, improved survival. Alcohol excess or the co-existence of other liver disease, such as fatty liver [non-alcoholic fatty liver (NAFL)], steatohepatitis (NASH), or chronic hepatitis C, accelerated liver damage.

Liver disease is typically silent. Symptoms may be absent, and physical signs of advancing damage and scarring (fibrosis) may be subtle or difficult to detect. Nonspecific symptoms, such as fatigue, loss of energy, aching of muscles and joints, weight loss, and abdominal discomfort, may not point to underlying liver disease. In the absence of any specific liver-related symptoms, diagnosing underlying liver disease depends upon blood test results (see Liver Blood Tests in Chapter 2).

CIRRHOSIS. Some people have symptoms that clearly point to advanced, cirrhotic-stage liver disease: swelling of ankles or abdomen, easy bruising or bleeding, yellowing of the whites of the eyes, poor concentrating ability, memory lapses, or periods of confusion. Occasionally, the symptoms include a noticeable enlargement of the liver, gastrointestinal hemorrhage, or a serious infection.

Jaundice and Other Signs. The most obvious sign of cirrhosis is jaundice, yellowing of the skin and whites (sclerae) of the eyes. Jaundice occurs with the accumulation of bilirubin, a chemical in the body that is normally eliminated by the liver through the bile.

When a doctor examines you, he also may find enlargement of the liver and spleen, abnormal liver tests, dilated capillaries of the skin (spider telangiectasia), reddening of the palms of the hands, easy bruising, fluid accumulation in the ankles and abdomen, and mental alterations.

Increasing jaundice and progressive increase in the other findings indicate worsening of liver disease.

During my jaundiced period, I looked like French vanilla ice cream. The whites of my eyes were yellow. My skin was a pale yellow.

ROY

How do iron overload and liver damage cause the signs and symptoms of HH? As liver disease progresses, fibrous tissue accumulates. This causes cirrhosis, which distorts the architecture of the liver and impairs the inflow of blood. The greater resistance to liver blood flow increases pressure within the portal vein. The resulting condition, portal hypertension, is associated with three obvious clinical features: ascites, varices, and encephalopathy.

Ascites and Edema. Ascites is the accumulation of fluid in the abdomen, causing abdominal swelling and weight gain. It results from chemical signals sent from the liver to the kidney that cause retention of salt and water. Because ascites is due to a generalized accumulation of fluid within the body, it is frequently associated with ankle swelling, also known as edema.

Doctors treat ascites and edema with salt restriction, diuretic medication, and, occasionally, a liver shunt, called a transjugular intrahepatic portal-systemic shunt (TIPS). Radiologists place the TIPS by puncturing a vein in the neck and positioning a catheter into the large veins that drain the liver. They fashion a channel within the liver to connect the portal vein to the hepatic veins. The TIPS shunt is placed within this channel, relieving the high pressure in the portal vein. As a result, ascites fluid is resorbed, and the abdominal distention resolves.

Varices. Varices, large veins within the esophagus and stomach, develop due to the redirection of portal blood flow away from the liver. You are unaware of varices until they bleed, or until they are detected by direct visualization of the esophagus by radiologic studies or endoscopic procedures.

One-and-a-half years ago, I had an incident where I was bleeding out. The varices in my esophagus just popped, I guess, so I lost a lot of blood. I was extremely anemic with a hematocrit in the low 20s. So my regular doctor prescribed iron supplements.

It was not pleasant. Taking iron is hard on your stomach. A month later, I found out from a hepatologist that I had excess iron because of hemochromatosis. I put the iron in irony because of that prescription for iron pills. Now I'm on the liver transplant waiting list.

RICHARD

Gastrointestinal hemorrhage from varices is dramatic, with patients vomiting large amounts of bright red blood or passing dark, maroon feces. Often, the bleeding is a medical emergency and is associated with a drop in blood pressure, rapid heart rate, and sweating. The risk of bleeding from varices is proportional to the severity of the portal hypertension. Doctors treat varices with medications, endoscopic procedures (sclerotherapy, band ligation), or TIPS.

Encephalopathy. Encephalopathy is the altered mental function and disordered mood or psychological status related to the buildup of ammonia and other chemicals from impaired liver metabolism. Early changes of encephalopathy may consist only of mental slowing, changes in memory, or mild impairment of complex tasks. More severe grades of encephalopathy are characterized by episodes of confusion, agitation, mood alteration, psychiatric symptoms, hallucinations, and even coma.

I didn't know I had hemochromatosis. I had never heard of it. Christmas eve, I was shopping with my boys. I was trying to walk faster to keep up with them, but I got slower. I thought I had the flu. I went home and got in bed. I opened Christmas presents, and I vaguely remember being on a couch.

The next day, I didn't recognize members of my family. They took me to the emergency room. Three days later, I woke up and didn't know where I was. I had gone into a coma because the poisons from my liver went to my brain, and my brain shut down.

SIMON

Other factors often precipitate bouts of encephalopathy, such as gastrointestinal bleeding, infection, dehydration, or electrolyte imbalance. Encephalopathy is usually treated with lactulose or the non-absorbable antibiotic, neomycin. In severe cases, protein restriction may be necessary.

Impairment of Synthetic and Metabolic Functions. Cirrhosis can lead to the impairment of the synthetic and metabolic functions of the liver. The liver manufactures many critical proteins necessary for the body's normal functioning, including clotting factors, albumin, hormone binding proteins, vitamin binding proteins, proteins for transporting lipids, and many others. A reduced synthesis of clotting factors increases the risk of bleeding or bruising easily with minor trauma. A low albumin level promotes water and salt retention, ascites, and edema.

The liver is integrally involved in the metabolism of ammonia, lipids, hormones, cholesterol, vitamins, proteins, and carbohydrates. The inability to detoxify ammonia promotes encephalopathy, and the disordered metabolism of hormones may cause impotence, sexual dysfunction, and feminization in men. Features of the latter can include breast enlargement, the loss of secondary sexual characteristics, and the emergence of telangiectasia (small vessels and capillaries in a spider-like pattern) in the skin.

In addition, impaired metabolism reduces the ability to detoxify or eliminate medications, drugs, or toxins from the body. Patients with cirrhosis typically require reduction in doses because they are "overly sensitive" to standard regimens of medications.

Signs and Symptoms Due to the Involvement of Other Organs

HEART. Iron accumulates in the muscle cells of the heart in untreated hemochromatosis. From 6 to 33 percent of HH patients may die of complications of heart failure or arrhythmia as iron accumulation degenerates heart muscle. This complication tends to occur in patients with highly accelerated iron accumulation who have clinical signs of HH in late adolescence or early adult life.

> In 1993, I started having heart palpitations, and I was fatigued all the time. My doctor did a liver biopsy and found that all that was left functioning of my liver was 10 to 15 percent. I had over a pound of iron in my liver.

> One symptom I did have before diagnosis was an irregular heartbeat. Ever since I've been de-ironed, I don't have it.

Cardiac involvement might be signaled by enlargement of the heart on a chest radiograph or minor changes in an electrocardiogram. When cardiac disease progresses, fluid may accumulate in the lungs (pulmonary edema) or in the rest of the body, including the ankles (peripheral edema). A heart biopsy, although rarely indicated, will reveal iron accumulation in the muscle cells with the degeneration of cells, but with little or no inflammation or fibrosis.

Cardiac dysfunction, particularly at early stages, may be reversed by the removal of body iron with phlebotomy. Echocardiographic studies of small numbers of patients have demonstrated improvement in cardiac function after removal of 2 to 18 grams of iron by phlebotomy. Severe, advanced cardiac disease may not respond but may require additional therapies, including heart transplantation. Some studies suggest that homozygosity and heterozygosity for HH may increase risk for coronary artery disease, although other studies fail to demonstrate a relationship.

PANCREAS. Iron accumulates in specialized insulin-producing cells of the pancreas called islet cells. With time, islet cells become irreversibly damaged and destroyed; insulin levels drop, rendering the patient diabetic.

> *I went to the doctor thinking I had a urinary tract infection. The internist did a urinalysis. Then a nurse came in and said, "Have you ever been tested for diabetes?"*
> *I'll be on insulin for the rest of my life.*

> *Periodically, my husband would have high glucose readings. We'd be in a store, and he'd collapse, disoriented. We didn't know if it was a seizure or what.*
> *Looking back, I think it was low sugar, because we now know he has hard-to-control, brittle diabetes. He takes insulin about four times a day. It's a pain in the neck.*

Symptoms of diabetes mellitus might include excessive thirst, excessive urination, waking in the middle of the night to urinate, or weight loss. Diabetes is irreversible and requires insulin therapy.

ENDOCRINE SYSTEM. The major endocrine function impaired by iron overload is insulin production by the islets, leading to diabetes mellitus. The next most common endocrine disorder relates to the reproductive system. I have already mentioned that impaired metabolism due to liver dysfunction can alter female and male hormones and contribute to impotence and sexual dysfunction. In addition, iron overload within pituitary gland or ovaries and testes can directly impair gonadal hormone production, further compromising reproductive and sexual function.

Hormonal production by gonads is controlled by other hormones (gonadotrophins, FSH, LH) secreted from the pituitary gland, located in the brain. Iron accumulates in specific cells of the anterior pituitary that are responsible for the production of the regulatory hormones and reduces the production of female (estrogen, progesterone) and male (testerone) steroid hormones from the ovary and testis, respectively.

> *My first real symptom was very obvious—a decline in sexual function—the ability to get and keep an erection. A year before, I had been a raging man. Then this happened, and I was really puzzled. I tried ginseng, but it had no effect.*
>
> *At my yearly physical, I mentioned it to my doctor, who ordered blood tests. My liver function was out of whack; the bilirubin was over the limit. He thought I had hepatitis. That test came back negative. But man, my ferritin was greater than 1,000.*
>
> *The doctor said I had hemochromatosis. I was the first case he ever diagnosed.*

> *At age 29, my menstrual cycle stopped, and I started having hot flashes. Countless doctors said it couldn't be menopause, that I was too young. Finally, I found one doctor who did a laparoscopy. He actually looked at the ovaries and found that they were shriveled and dried up. We still didn't have an answer, but he determined that I had gone into premature menopause.*
>
> *Normally, I would have shed blood at the end of the month, but I quit doing that so I was storing more and more iron. I started feeling very tired. Over a period of two years, several doctors said I was probably anemic and should take more iron. I felt terrible.*
>
> *It took nine years—until I was 38—before a gastroenterologist diagnosed me with hemochromatosis. He did a liver biopsy, and I had some cirrhosis. I did weekly phlebotomies for eighteen months. It took almost a year before we saw my ferritin levels go down to 10 or 12.*
>
> *My gastroenterologist said, "I can tell you what happened to your ovaries. That was the first thing the iron destroyed."*

My husband's glands were affected. Everything was low—his thyroid, pituitary. He tried cortisone, and he was taking testosterone for a while. He took meds for all those things. Seemed like he was deficient in everything.

Nine years after I was diagnosed, I remarried. I had lost the ability to get an erection, but I wanted to get sexually active again so I went to the doctor to try to restore this function. I tried papavarin, which is injected into the shaft with a needle, and a suction device that didn't work. The only thing that seemed possible was an implant in the penis. Then my wife's physical ability declined because of multiple sclerosis— so the need kind of went away.

As iron stores in various organs of the body, it apparently can damage the pituitary, which regulates testosterone. I tried testosterone shots, but they weren't effective, and they can have side effects. When all my attempts failed, the urologist said he didn't have good success with HH patients and erectile dysfunction.

I recently went to see him again, and he gave me a sample of Viagra. I haven't tried it yet.

SKIN. Iron deposits in the skin increase pigmentation to produce a bronze appearance. Historically, "bronze diabetes" was another term used to describe patients with hemochromatosis, highlighting the relationship between iron overload, increased pigmentation of the skin, and diabetes mellitus.

No one ever said anything about my bronzing, but it was noticeable to me. I work inside all day, but I look like I work outside.

Since I was a teenager, I've had bronzed skin. I thought it was because I am part Indian. Everyone wanted to know how I kept my tan all year round.

The bronzing gradually faded when I was de-ironed. I'm very pale now. And I was always so proud of my Indian heritage. My grandfather was a full-blooded Cherokee.

BONES AND JOINTS. Bone thinning (osteoporosis, osteopenia) is common and increases the risk of fractures. Approximately 50 percent of patients with hemochromatosis complain of joint pain and exhibit arthritic changes on radiographic evaluation.

> When I turned 60, I went from fine to horrible in three months. I couldn't walk, and I had my left hip replaced. A year later, my right hip started twinging. It scared me to death.
>
> I went to a rheumatologist and asked him to look at my osteoarthritis. He asked me which joints in my hands hurt, and I said all of them.
>
> "Even the big knuckles?" he asked. "You don't have rheumatoid arthritis, and it's not just osteoarthritis. I think I know what it is—hemochromatosis."
>
> He X-rayed my hands and feet and saw big changes. "That's why your hip went," he said.
>
> My doctor is a god. Other physicians hear hoof beats outside the tent and say it's horses; my doctor looks for zebras.

> A doctor came to my HH support group. He said a telltale sign of HH is arthritis in the hands and the swelling of the knuckles where the fingers meet the hand. Well, my hand was swollen. I had almost no grip. If someone shook my hand real hard, I almost passed out from the pain.
>
> With phlebotomy, the swelling went down. It's not perfect. I have a pretty good grip but not much dexterity.

> My joints are pretty toasted.

> In 1990, I had a fall in my house and broke four toes. Did my bones actually break because they were getting thin from undiagnosed preosteoporosis? Or did I just have a bad fall. Some people blame every problem they've got on HH.

Joint involvement (arthritis) causes pain and swelling and characteristically affects the metacarpal-phalangeal joints, located between the hand and base of the fingers. The characteristic joints are the second and third joints, adjacent to the thumb, although the smaller joints of the fingers, knees, back, feet, hips, wrists, and shoulders may also be involved. Symptoms from joint involvement may be the first indicator of hemochromatosis; radiographs of the hands can be diagnostic.

INFECTION. Patients with hemochromatosis may be uniquely susceptible to infection by relatively unusual organisms including Vibrio vulnificus (cholera-like organism), Listeria (unusual cause of meningitis or infectious arthritis), Yersinia enterocolitica and Salmonella (diarrheal disease, biliary infection, hepatic abscess), Klebsiella, E coli, and fungi (Rhizopus and mucor species). Hemochromatosis should be suspected in any patient presenting with one of these infections.

Summary

Iron accumulation damages tissues and organs, impairing function and resulting in signs and symptoms of disease. The liver is the main storage depot for the excess iron, and liver disease dominates the clinical picture. Iron targets other organs and tissues, such as the heart, pancreas, joints, and pituitary, and leads to a myriad of additional signs and symptoms. However, not all medical illnesses occurring in patients with hemochromatosis can be attributed to iron overload. In this chapter we discussed clinical problems clearly associated with iron accumulation in specific organs.

Strike while the iron is hot.
RABELAIS

6

Taking Care of Yourself Nutritionally

Guidelines for Healthy Nutrition in Hemochromatosis

I eat more chicken and fish now, plus vegetables and salad. Potatoes are high iron. I love them, but I have to cut back. I try to minimize my intake of iron, because the more I take in, the more phlebotomies I have to have. I have a choice—so I choose to take in less iron.

On the other hand, iron is in everything that grows in the ground. You can't quit living. So I still eat meat and stuff but not the quantities I did before. I go toward the white meats rather than the red ones.

JIM

MANY PEOPLE, WHEN THEY DISCOVER THEY have hereditary hemochromatosis, ask about an iron-free or iron-reduced diet. It's a natural question, but no type of diet can completely control iron overload, because iron is in almost everything we eat. If we cut out iron, we also cut out other nutrients our bodies need.

An estimated 10 percent of iron in our food is available for absorption by our bodies. A normal metabolism allows the body to absorb about 1 milligram of iron a day to replace the same amount that is routinely lost through the sloughing of dead skin and gut cells, and the growth of fingernails and hair. The metabolism of a person with HH, however, allows the body to absorb too much iron. And once absorbed, the iron has no way to be naturally discarded.

To safely reduce iron, you must maintain the schedule of phlebotomy treatments your doctor prescribes. It is especially important for people on treatment to (1) eat properly in order to avoid anemia and (2) stay hydrated by drinking sufficient fluids. With hemochromatosis, therefore, the goal is to eat a well-balanced, healthy diet.

CAUTION: If late-stage hemochromatosis has damaged body organs, consult your medical specialists about specific dietary measures. For example, people with heart problems or cirrhosis of the liver may require sodium restriction, while diabetics need to monitor sugar and carbohydrate intake. Always check with your doctor before making major changes in your diet or before taking over-the-counter supplements and vitamins.

In this chapter, I'll discuss dietary iron, nutritional "dos and don'ts" for people with hemochromatosis, an overview of a normal, well-balanced diet, nutrition and the liver, and dietary considerations for people with liver disease and cirrhosis:

- *Dietary Iron*
    - How Do We Absorb Iron?
- *Some Nutritional DOs and DON'Ts for People with Hemochromatosis*
    - The DOs
    - The DON'Ts
- *Nutrition Tips from Patients*
- *Nutritional Overview*
    - Ideal Body Weight
    - Normal Diet
- *Nutrition and the Liver*
    - Overview
    - Carbohydrate Metabolism
    - Protein Metabolism
    - Fat Metabolism
    - Bile

VITAMINS
- *Nutritional Needs for Hemochromatosis Patients with Liver Disease but without Cirrhosis*
  CALORIC REQUIREMENTS
  VITAMIN SUPPLEMENTS
- *Nutritional Needs for Hemochromatosis Patients with Cirrhosis*
  CALORIC REQUIREMENTS
  PROTEIN RESTRICTION
  VITAMIN SUPPLEMENTS
  MINERAL SUPPLEMENTS
  SALT AND FLUID RESTRICTION

Dietary Iron

Iron is a nutrient found in our diets. Red meat, for example, contains highly absorbable iron, while plants (such as grains, nuts, vegetables, and fruits) contain less easily absorbed iron. If you have hemochromatosis, you may absorb two to three times the amount of iron from meat than you would if you had normal metabolism.

I would like to emphasize that attempts to reduce dietary iron do not replace the prescribed phlebotomy treatments. Work with your physician to maintain a phlebotomy regimen that's right for you as well as a healthy, balanced diet (see Nutritional Overview, below).

Nevertheless, you may decide that it's helpful (and healthful) to reduce the amount of iron in your diet. Certain foods, such as calcium and tea, tend to decrease the absorption of iron. Other substances, such as vitamin C, tend to increase iron absorption (see the list of dietary Dos and Don'ts below).

RESOURCE: Garrison, Cheryl. *Cooking with Less Iron.* Nashville: Cumberland House, 2001. This book offers detailed dietary information, food composition charts, menu planners, sample menus, and recipes for people with iron overload.

HOW DO WE ABSORB IRON? The mechanisms of absorption of iron from the gut into the intestinal blood circulation are complex and not completely understood. Nonetheless, researchers have described many of the basic processes and have defined much of the molecular basis for iron absorption.

Dietary iron exists in two primary forms: elemental iron and heme iron. Elemental iron has two forms, ferric and ferrous iron. Ferric iron (Fe^{+3}), the predominant form of dietary iron, must be reduced to ferrous iron (Fe^{+2}) prior to transport by specific membrane proteins in the plasma membrane of cells lining the duodenum (DMT1).

The conversion of ferric to ferrous iron is accomplished by an enzyme (ferrireductase) in the duodenal lining cells and facilitated by the gastric secretion of acid and proteins. The activity of the transport protein, DMT1, is programmed by the degree of total body iron. The activity of DMT1 is low when body iron is high, and the activity of DMT1 is high when body iron is low. In contrast, intestinal lining cells absorb heme iron by a different pathway.

In hereditary hemochromatosis, the pathways for absorption of iron do not respond to increases in body iron stores. The HFE mutation produces a protein that disrupts the normal regulatory pathways of iron absorption by the intestinal lining cells. As a result, iron absorption continues at an increased rate despite the accumulation of total body iron.

Once iron enters the intestinal lining cell, it has one of two fates. It is either stored in the cell bound to the protein, ferritin, or it is transported out of the intestinal lining cell into the blood. Iron in blood is typically bound to a circulating transport protein, transferrin, and delivered via the circulation to cells of the body. The body's cells take up iron via an interaction between transferrin and a specific protein in the plasma membrane of cells, transferrin receptor.

Iron is stored in the body's cells in the form of cell-bound ferritin or hemosiderin. Iron leaves the body through blood loss (menstruation, pregnancy, bleeding) or the sloughing of skin and gut lining cells, fingernails or hair.

Some Nutritional DOs and DON'Ts for People with Hemochromatosis

THE DOs
DO eat a balanced diet.

DO stay well-hydrated. Drinking plenty of fluids (2 to 2 1/2 quarts per day) is desirable but is especially important before and after phlebotomy treatments. Hydration will reduce the time it takes to remove blood.

DO read food labels. Since 1990, when the Nutritional Labeling and Education Act was passed, all food products in the United States display labels that include iron content. Remember, however, that this is the amount of iron in the food, not the amount of iron your body absorbs.

Once you get in the habit of reading labels, you'll be surprised at how many foods contain iron. Look for ingredients that begin with the Latin word for iron (ferrum) or the chemical symbol for iron (Fe). For example, you may see ferrous sulfate, ferrous fulmate, ferrous gluconate or ferrochel.

Choose breakfast cereals, breads, or pastas that are not fortified or "enriched" with iron. Read labels carefully. One serving of Old Fashioned Quaker Oats, for example, contains 10 percent of daily iron values, while the regular flavor of Quaker Instant Oatmeal contains 45 percent.

DO eat your fruits and vegetables. The iron in fruits, vegetables, nuts, and grain is less easily absorbed by the body than animal-based iron.

DO reduce your intake of red meat. Red meat is a high source of iron in a form readily absorbed by the body. You don't have to eliminate meat (it's a good source of vitamin B). Simply eat it less often and in smaller portions.

DO drink apple juice and tea. Apple juice is believed to inhibit iron absorption. The tannin in regular black teas (not herbal teas) is also thought to have the same effect.

DO check the iron content of your water supply if you are drinking well water, which is high in iron.

DO consider taking a vitamin B complex (including B6 acid or folate and B12) if you are on phlebotomy treatment—after you check with your doctor, of course.

DO talk to your doctor about hepatitis A and hepatitis B vaccinations. These preventable infections can be dangerous for people with liver disease and hemochromatosis.

THE DON'Ts

DON'T drink alcohol. Alcohol enhances iron absorption and hastens liver disease. Alcohol causes liver damage, and iron overload from hemochromatosis causes liver damage. The damage from both together is more than additive.

Don't drink at all or at least abstain until you finish your initial phlebotomy treatments and your liver enzymes are normal. If you return to social drinking, limit your consumption to less than 2 ounces per week.

DON'T smoke. Tobacco smoke is high in iron.

DON'T take iron pills or a daily multivitamin with iron. Look for a daily multivitamin brand, such as Centrum Silver, that doesn't contain iron.

DON'T take any prescription or over-the-counter medicines without checking labels for iron content and without clearing them with your doctor. Seemingly innocuous products can contain iron.

DON'T take vitamin C supplements. Vitamin C supplements bind with iron in a way that increases iron absorption. It is difficult, if not impossible, to find a multivitamin without vitamin C, but look for a limited intake of 500 milligrams or less per day.

Vitamin C naturally occurs in fruits and vegetables. One glass of juice a day fulfills your body's need for vitamin C. There is little evidence to support use of high doses of vitamin C, and this practice is to be discouraged, especially in patients with hemochromatosis.

DON'T forget to check processed food labels for added vitamin C as well as iron.

DON'T take vitamin C-rich juices or supplements 24 hours before you get tested for iron levels.

DON'T use cast-iron skillets for cooking.

DON'T diet to lose weight while on phlebotomy treatment.

DON'T eat or handle raw shellfish, such as oysters or clams. Cooked seafood and fish are fine. Raw or partially cooked molluscan shellfish can be infected with marine bacteria, particularly Vibrio species, such as vulnificus, which can be especially toxic to people with liver disease and hemochromatosis.

RESOURCE: For more information, call the Food and Drug Administration hotline: 1-888-SAFEFOOD or access the FDA Web site at www.fda.gov and search for "seafood hemochromatosis." The FDA's Center for Food Safety and Applied Nutrition, Consumer Education Staff, is located at HFS-555, 200 C St. S.W., Washington, DC 20204.

Nutrition Tips from Patients

People with hemochromatosis find varied ways to reduce dietary iron and to work toward healthier eating habits. Here are some of their suggestions:

I'm a firm believer in regulating iron intake in my diet, although other people don't think it's that important. I think that's the reason why I need phlebotomies only every six months.

In my opinion, you can go crazy watching your food for iron. If you and your doctor are serious about keeping your iron down, one phlebotomy session will be as effective as maybe a year of watching your diet. I eat anything I want and I control my iron by phlebotomies.

My theory is any extra iron is too much iron. I eat egg yolks only occasionally. I pretty much stick to chicken, turkey, and fish; they're the lowest in iron.

Sadly for me, one of my favorite foods is liver and onions—and spinach. Both are high in iron. So I don't eat liver at all, and I very seldom eat red meat.

I try to eat a balanced diet with a lowered iron intake. Animal liver is the highest natural source of iron. I love liver. But maybe I'll have it three times a year, not once a month.

They tell you right away to avoid iron—dark greens like spinach, organs like liver, and cereals fortified with iron. I was pretty rigid at the beginning. I love seafood so I ate that.

As soon as I got my iron levels down, I asked my doctor about prime rib. He said once a week wouldn't bother me—just don't eat it regularly.

I'm a vegetarian. I like spinach and green, leafy vegetables. Now I have to watch out because they're all high in iron.

When my dad found out he had hemochromatosis, he said, "Stay away from iron. Don't even cook in an iron wok. Don't eat tomatoes or cereals high in iron."

I had a lovely set of cast-iron skillets. My doctor said, "You don't want to cook with those." Iron leaches into the food.

I don't eat bacon, eggs, and orange juice together because the vitamin C in the juice increases iron absorption. I drink tea, because caffeine inhibits the body's ability to absorb iron. I take a multiple vitamin with no iron, and I look for breakfast cereals with the least amount of iron.

I never liked orange juice, which is good because you want to monitor your vitamin C. But I drink a pot of tea a day—at least five cups.

I don't have diabetes, but I've been following a diabetic diet, and exercising, to balance my endocrine system. That means no sugar. (Well, sometimes I have a cookie.)

I monitor my carbohydrates. I try to stay as iron deficient as possible by eating high protein, like legumes, minimal starches, and I try not to have carbohydrates unless they come from vegetables or fruit. Green beans, for example, have 2.7 grams of carbs. That's good. Corn is high in carbs—not good.

When I was growing up, I used to go through three pints of milk a day. Later, I learned that calcium inhibits iron absorption.

I was such a cheese freak that my dad would say, "Did you park the cow out back?"

I have a friend with HH, and one of the pleasures of his day was having a glass of wine with dinner. His doctor told him he had to watch his diet and give up wine altogether.

But from what I learned, I knew he really didn't have to do that if he was having periodic phlebotomies. It's a quality of life issue. If you love liver and onions, have it once in a while. Just make sure your iron is monitored.

Egg yolks are heavy in iron so I have bacon and eggs every third day. I love eggs, but they're not encouraged because of cholesterol. However, my doctor said I have low cholesterol, and that's one of the bennies of hemochromatosis.

Before I got in trouble, I used to take a one-a-day vitamin with iron. I don't do that anymore!

I like bran flakes. The lowest iron content I've found is 25 percent. I buy that. Raisins have a lot of iron, so raisin bran is high in iron. I pick out a lot of the raisins, because I like the taste of that kind of bran more. But raisins are one of my snack foods. I just refuse to be extreme in my dieting. I don't want to give up the foods I like.

Iron-fortified cereals are dangerous. It's like eating rust.

I've never found a popular commercial cold cereal with less than 25 percent D.V. (Daily Value) of iron, except for something like shredded wheat. I buy Irish Oatmeal; it's got 6 percent D.V. and takes a half hour to cook.
I prepare about 4 to 6 portions at once, which have the consistency of rubber. Then I put the portions in a plastic bag and refrigerate them. This lasts me a week or two. I just warm them up in the microwave.

Now you can find natural cereals that don't use additives so there's no iron. I love oatmeal and shredded wheat, and they're low iron. Remember! Avoid the word "fortified." It means iron.

I want to have cereal so I modify my wife's granola recipe by taking out anything fortified with iron. Then I put shredded wheat biscuits in a bowl and add my granola. This way I get the taste and texture of granola plus a lot of fiber. I call it Hemochromatosis Granola:
Preheat oven to 350°F. Grease two baking sheets. In a large bowl combine:
18-ounce box Old Fashioned Quaker Oats
1 cup shredded coconut
1 cup wheat bran (wheat germ is an alternative but it has some iron)

3/4 *cup slivered almonds*
1/2 *cup raw sunflower seeds*

In a medium bowl mix together and combine well:
1/2 *cup water*
1 1/2 *teaspoons salt*
1 1/2 *teaspoons vanilla extract*

To the water and salt mixture add:
1/2 *cup honey*
1/2 *cup cooking oil*

Pour the wet ingredients over the dry and mix well. Divide mixture between the 2 prepared baking sheets, spreading evenly and to the edges to prevent burning. Bake for 10 minutes. Remove baking sheets from oven and stir the granola. Return to the oven and bake 10 minutes more. Remove from oven and stir again. Return to oven for 10 minutes or so until browned to satisfaction. Check frequently to make sure granola doesn't burn.

I bag mine in a reclosable plastic bag and keep it in the refrigerator. Enjoy!

Nutritional Overview

IDEAL BODY WEIGHT. Most people worry about their weight with good reason. One in three American adults is overweight, a statistic that's up from one in four only a decade ago.

What, then, should you weigh? We have no exact measure of ideal body weight because the "norm" is based on population statistics, cultural perceptions, and the influence of genetically and environmentally determined differences in metabolism. In short, there are no absolute rules, only working guidelines:

- ◆ **MEN:** 106 pounds for the first five feet, then add six pounds for every inch thereafter
- ◆ **WOMEN:** 100 pounds for the first five feet, then add five pounds for every inch thereafter

Remember, do not diet to lose weight if you are on protocol phlebotomy treatments. When you lose weight, you typically lose a relatively greater amount of fluid and become relatively dehydrated. If you are dehydrated at the time of phlebotomy it may be more difficult for the phlebotomist to place the needle in your vein. In addition, when blood is withdrawn, you would be more prone to a drop in blood pressure and fainting.

NORMAL DIET. Food supplies us with carbohydrates, fats, and proteins that in turn supply energy. Energy is measured in calories. Carbohydrates and proteins provide approximately 4 calories per gram, and fat provides almost 9 calories per gram—twice as much. People also need essential nutrients (such as certain vitamins, minerals, amino acids, and fatty acids) and other substances, such as fiber, from a variety of foods. Oranges, for example, are rich in vitamin C, bananas supply potassium, and a half-cup serving of cantaloupe contributes half of the daily requirement for beta-carotene. A normal, healthy diet contains the amounts of essential nutrients and calories you need to prevent either a nutritional deficiency or excess and provides the right balance of carbohydrate, fat, and protein.

Many Americans, however, don't have good eating habits. According to the Healthy Eating Index of the U.S. Department of Agriculture (USDA) Center for Nutrition Policy and Promotion, only about 17 percent of people eat the recommended number of servings of fruit, and only about 31 percent eat the recommended number of servings of vegetables. In fact, diet-related health conditions (heart disease, stroke, cancer, and diabetes) "cost society about $250 billion annually in medical costs and lost productivity. 30 to 40 percent of deaths due to cancer can be prevented if people will choose a healthful diet and perform physical activity."[1]

What is a healthful diet? The USDA currently recommends a daily caloric intake of 30 to 40 calories per kilogram of body weight and the following dietary balance:

- *40 to 50 percent carbohydrate*
- *No more than 30 percent fat (less than 10 percent of calories from saturated fat)*
- *1 to 1.5 grams of protein for each kilogram (2.2 lbs.) of body weight*

For more information about healthy diets, I recommend you consult the Food Guide Pyramid published by the USDA. It graphically illustrates the importance of balance among different food groups in a daily

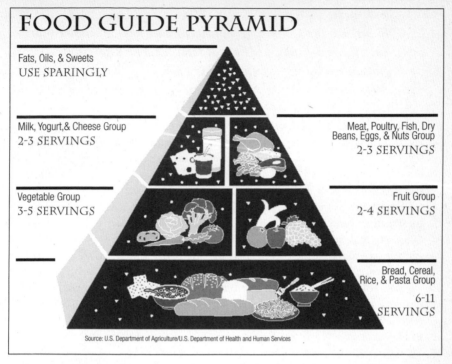

FOOD GUIDE PYRAMID

Fats, Oils, & Sweets
USE SPARINGLY

Milk, Yogurt,& Cheese Group
2-3 SERVINGS

Meat, Poultry, Fish, Dry
Beans, Eggs, & Nuts Group
2-3 SERVINGS

Vegetable Group
3-5 SERVINGS

Fruit Group
2-4 SERVINGS

Bread, Cereal,
Rice, & Pasta Group
6-11
SERVINGS

Source: U.S. Department of Agriculture/U.S. Department of Health and Human Services

eating pattern and suggests the number (depending on daily calorie intake desired) and size of daily servings. As you can see, you should choose a variety of grains (especially whole grains lacking fortification with iron), fruits, and vegetables.

Pyramid serving sizes are not large. For example, 1 serving equals 1/2 cup of pasta; 1 cup of raw, leafy vegetables; 1/2 cup of other vegetables (cooked or chopped raw); 1 medium apple, banana, orange; 1 cup of milk or yogurt; or 2 to 3 ounces of cooked lean meat, poultry, or fish.

The USDA recommendations include a range of servings from each of the five major food groups. People who consume about 1,600 calories a day should be guided by the smaller number; the larger number is for people who are very active and consume about 2,800 calories a day:

- *Choose most of your daily foods from the bread, cereal, rice, and pasta group (6–11 servings), vegetable group (3–5 servings), and fruit group (2–4 servings). Remember to choose non- or low-iron fortified or enriched breads, cereals, and pasta.*
- *Choose moderate amounts of foods from the milk, yogurt, and cheese group (2–3 servings) and the meat, poultry, fish, dry beans, eggs, and nuts group (2–3 servings).*
- *Limit foods that provide few nutrients and are high in fat*

and sugar.

♦ *In general, the USDA recommends a diet low in saturated fat and cholesterol and moderate in total fat. The new 2000 guidelines also urge you to choose appropriate beverages and foods in order to moderate your intake of sugars and salt.*

RESOURCE: To buy copies of *Dietary Guidelines for Americans* and *Using the Dietary Guidelines for Americans*, call the Federal Consumer Information Center toll-free: 1-888-878-3256 or download nutritional material, including the Food Guide Pyramid, from the USDA Center for Nutrition Policy and Promotion Web site at www.usda.gov/cnpp

RESOURCE: The American Dietetic Association's (ADA) Nutrition Information Line (to find qualified dieticians in your area) is 1-800-366-1655. Helpful books: *Complete Food & Nutrition Guide* by Roberta Duyff and the ADA and *Dieting for Dummies* by Jane Kirby and the ADA. Web site: www.eatright.org

RESOURCE: The American Institute for Cancer Research provides practical tips on good nutrition with its newsletter, pamphlets, and a toll-free AICR Nutrition Hotline staffed by a registered dietician: Call 1-800-843-8114 and ask for Nutrition Information. Web site: www.aicr.org

RESOURCE: *Nutrition Action Newsletter* (Center for Science in the Public Interest). Web site: www.cspinet.org

RESOURCE: Learn about your "5 a day" minimum number of fruits and vegetables for a healthy diet, recipes, and tips for a healthy lifestyle. Web site: www.5aday.gov/

Nutrition and Your Liver

OVERVIEW. The liver is your body's major digestive organ. When the liver receives nutrients from the intestines, it metabolizes*, packages, stores, and sends them to other organs where they are used for energy. Your liver's major nutritional jobs include:

♦ *Metabolizing carbohydrates, proteins, and fat for energy*
♦ *Assimilating and storing vitamins*
♦ *Manufacturing bile to aid in digestion and absorption of fats*
♦ *Filtering and destroying toxins (including alcohol and drugs)*

Throughout this chapter we use the term "metabolism," which we define as the body processes, including a whole host of chemical reactions that are necessary to maintain function and sustain life.

The liver is the major organ responsible for regulating and responding to your body's metabolic demands. Your liver must be functioning well to maintain normal metabolism of carbohydrates, fats, and protein; it is also responsible for processing and using several vitamins. This section deals with the role a healthy liver (and a healthy, well-balanced diet) plays in these nutritional processes.

CARBOHYDRATE METABOLISM. The most common sources of dietary carbohydrates are sugars, such as sucrose (table sugar), fructose (corn syrup), and lactose (milk sugar); and starches, such as breads, pasta, grains, cereals, fruits, vegetables, and potatoes. When you eat carbohydrates, specialized enzymes in the pancreas and gut process them to yield simple sugars (glucose, galactose, fructose, maltose).

These sugars are absorbed by intestinal lining cells, enter the portal circulation, and travel to the liver via the portal vein. During overnight fasting, blood sugar levels dip to a relatively low level, insulin secretion is suppressed, and blood insulin levels diminish. After a meal, blood sugar increases (stimulating the release of insulin from the pancreas), and insulin levels rise. Insulin, which rises in response to a meal, is the hormone that stimulates the liver to take in more glucose and to move the glucose into storage—mainly in the form of glycogen. The liver can then release glycogen to your muscles for energy during periods of fasting or exercise.

Although the liver can store considerable amounts of glycogen, it is the first energy source used during periods of prolonged fasting or caloric deprivation, and it can be depleted rapidly. After glycogen, the body taps other energy sources—including protein and fat.

PROTEIN METABOLISM. We take in dietary protein from dairy products, produce, and meats. Enzymes produced by the pancreas and intestine break down the protein into its amino acids and small peptides. The intestine rapidly absorbs the amino acids with specific transport systems within its lining cells and then delivers the amino acids to the liver via the portal vein.

When they reach the liver, they are used for energy or for making (synthesizing) new proteins. The newly synthesized proteins perform specific body functions (see Table 6).

TABLE 6. SOME COMMON LIVER PROTEINS AND THEIR
         FUNCTION IN THE HUMAN BODY

Protein	Function
Clotting Factors (II, V, VII, IX, and X)	Maintain normal clotting
Albumin	Maintain normal blood volume
Renin	Regulate blood pressure
Binding globulins	Regulate hormone action
Transferrin	Transport iron
Ferritin	Store iron
Retinol binding protein	Transport Vitamin A to the eye
LDL receptor	Remove Cholesterol from the blood
P-450 proteins	Metabolize drugs, chemicals, toxins

FAT METABOLISM. In general, fats are neutral lipids (triglycerides), acidic lipids (fatty acids), and sterols (cholesterol, plant sterols). Triglycerides (dairy products, meats, oils, butter, margarine) are the most common type of dietary fat and represent a major source of energy. The liver is uniquely suited to regulate and process triglycerides.

Dietary triglyceride is digested in the intestine by lipase, an enzyme secreted by the pancreas in response to meals. Bile, secreted by the liver, makes the digested fat soluble and promotes its absorption. Absorbed fat is then repackaged and transported into blood, where the liver ultimately removes it from circulation. Fat that reaches the liver is processed in three ways: (1) stored as fat droplets in liver cells; (2) metabolized as a source of energy; and (3) repackaged, secreted back into blood, and delivered to other cells in the body.

The liver is also intimately involved with the processing of dietary cholesterol and is the main source of newly synthesized cholesterol in the body. Liver disease may be associated with both high or low blood cholesterol levels.

BILE. The liver produces and secretes a fluid (bile) that enters the intestine to aid in digestion and absorption. Bile is clear yellow to golden-brown and contains water, electrolytes (salts), cholesterol, bile salts (detergents), phospholipids, and proteins. Bile helps to activate enzymes secreted by the pancreas and is essential for the digestion and absorption of fat or fat-soluble vitamins.

TAKING CARE OF YOURSELF NUTRITIONALLY 93

VITAMINS. The liver plays a role in several steps of vitamin metabolism. I'll describe only a few of those steps. Vitamins are either fat-soluble (vitamins A, D, E, and K) or water-soluble (vitamin C and the B-complex vitamins).

Patients with advanced liver disease may become deficient in water-soluble vitamins, but this is usually due to inadequate nutrition and poor food intake. Vitamin B12 storage usually far exceeds the body's requirements; deficiencies rarely occur due to liver disease or liver failure. When dietary intake drops, however, thiamine and folate commonly become deficient. Oral supplementation is usually all that you need to restore thiamine and folate stores to the normal range.

Fat-soluble vitamins require not only adequate dietary intake but also good digestion and absorption by the body. That's why normal production of bile is essential. Bile in the gut is required for the absorption of fat-soluble vitamins into the body because these vitamins are relatively insoluble in water. Bile acts as a detergent, breaking down and dissolving these vitamins so they may be properly absorbed.

If bile production is poor, oral supplementation of vitamins A, D, E, and K may not be sufficient to restore vitamin levels to normal. The use of a detergent-like solution of liquid vitamin E (TPGS) improves the absorption of vitamin E in patients with advanced liver disease. The same solution may also improve the absorption of vitamins A, D, and K if the latter are taken simultaneously with the liquid vitamin E.

Nutritional Needs for Hemochromatosis Patients with Liver Disease but without Cirrhosis

CALORIC REQUIREMENTS. In general, the noncirrhotic patient has caloric needs similar to those of noninfected people of the same age and gender. For this reason we recommend the following:

- *No need for salt restriction*
- *No need for protein restriction*
- *30 to 40 calories per kilogram intake per day*
- *One multivitamin (without iron) per day*

Patients who drink excessive amounts of alcohol should stop drinking altogether. They may also need supplementation with thiamine and folate.

Patients often proudly tell me that they are restricting their protein intake to "help" their livers. I'd like to emphasize that moderate amounts of protein (as recommended by the Food Pyramid) should be a normal part of your diet. If you are concerned about fat content, choose low-fat sources of protein. Protein restriction is recommended only for patients with cirrhosis who have encephalopathy (mental confusion).

Common questions I'm asked are, "Will dietary fat harm my liver? Should I avoid fat? Can I digest fat?" Dietary fat (triglycerides) undergoes complex processing. In the setting of liver disease, fat may accumulate in the liver. However, dietary fat intake does not correlate with the degree of fatty accumulation. Nonetheless, liver fat (steatosis) may promote liver injury and fibrosis in patients. Therefore, we do recommend a diet relatively low in fat, particularly saturated fat.

On the other hand, hemochromatosis by itself does not alter fat digestion or absorption from the gut. Only patients with advanced liver disease (cirrhosis) with jaundice have altered fat digestion and absorption. Jaundice in the setting of cirrhosis indicates severe impairment of processing and secretion of bile. Reduced bile concentration in the gut limits fat digestion and absorption.

VITAMIN SUPPLEMENTS. In general, noncirrhotic patients with liver disease and hemochromatosis require no additional vitamin supplementation other than one multivitamin without iron per day. One theory of the development of liver disease is that oxidant stress promotes liver cell injury and also stimulates specialized cells in the liver (stellate cells) to produce the main fibrosis protein, collagen. Iron is a catalyst for oxidant injury by promoting formation of "free radicals" that can initiate injury and fibrosis.

Supplemental vitamin C may be of potential benefit because it has anti-oxidant properties. However, vitamin C may promote iron absorption and lead to excessive accumulation of iron in the liver. The latter effect could actually increase oxidant injury. A reasonable, middle-ground approach is to take in the daily FDA-recommended amount of vitamin C (not more than 500 milligrams per day) and to avoid excessive supplementation.

Nutritional Needs for Hemochromatosis Patients with Cirrhosis

CALORIC REQUIREMENTS. In general, the patient with early-stage or compensated cirrhosis still requires 30 to 40 calories per kilogram a day.

You may need to alter your dietary habits to take in this number of calories, because as hemochromatosis progresses to cirrhosis, you may begin to experience loss of appetite, increasing fatigue, reduction in physical activity, and alteration of your sleep-wake pattern. People commonly complain of loss of exercise tolerance ("I'm just too pooped out to get my work done"). In addition, these changes often precipitate a sense of despondency, anxiety, or depression. It helps to develop both a pattern of meals that allows you to use your diet for maximum energy and a rest pattern that reduces prolonged periods of physical activity.

No nutritional prescription is right for every patient. You need to address your specific nutritional needs with your physician. In my experience, patients with hemochromatosis who develop compensated cirrhosis benefit by more frequent, smaller volume meals. Instead of one or two large meals, divide the equivalent amount of calories into four smaller meals. In addition, supplementation with one or two tablets of multivitamins is generally indicated, although the overall benefit is unclear. Despite this change in dietary habit, fatigue often persists. People benefit from "rest periods," usually 30 minutes or an hour in the mid-afternoon.

CAUTION: Please understand that advanced cirrhosis is associated with severe impairment of liver function and that specific dietary modifications may be necessary and could alter the general guidelines noted above. Your doctor may recommend a consultation with a dietician or provide you with a specific nutritional prescription.

PROTEIN RESTRICTION. It is important that the patient with cirrhosis take in enough protein to avoid excessive muscle wasting and energy depletion. However, if encephalopathy develops, a doctor might prescribe a "protein-restricted" diet.

Encephalopathy is the alteration or cloudiness of mental function. When the condition is severe, the patient becomes disoriented, confused, combative, or even comatose. Encephalopathy may also cause altered sleep-wake patterns, altered personality, and lack of motor coordination.

One factor contributing to these symptoms is dietary protein intake, so patients with any of the above symptoms may be placed on protein restrictions. This diet is usually not zero protein, but a reduced level of 20 to 60 grams per day. Often, the physician will use other treatments in conjunction with this diet, such as lactulose or neomycin.

VITAMIN SUPPLEMENTS. Most people, even those with cirrhosis, have adequate intake and storage of water-soluble vitamins (C, B complex). To be sure, I recommend the addition of two tablets of multivitamins low in iron each day (one in the morning and one in the evening).

Patients who excessively use or abuse alcohol risk becoming deficient in these vitamins, particularly thiamine and folate, and they may benefit from taking supplements. As I have emphasized before, the patient with hemochromatosis should avoid alcohol. Those who avoid alcohol probably won't require either supplement.

MINERAL SUPPLEMENTS. Patients with cirrhosis may experience deficiencies in three minerals: calcium, magnesium, and zinc. Calcium deficiency may be related to a lack of vitamin D, poor nutrition, or malabsorption. Correcting the underlying abnormality may be all that is required to restore calcium balance. However, bone thinning may occur even without these specific problems, so I recommend 0.5 to 1.0 grams of calcium each day. Calcium may be taken in the form of dairy products or therapeutic supplements. When the patient can't take in enough dairy products because of protein, salt, or fluid restrictions (see next section), supplements are used.

Magnesium deficiency may occur due to inadequate dietary intake. However, it occurs more often when patients take diuretics to treat fluid retention because their kidneys flush out the magnesium as waste. Symptoms of magnesium deficiency include muscle cramps, fatigue, weakness, nausea, and vomiting. Often, it's not possible to modify or discontinue diuretics in cirrhotic patients, so magnesium supplementation (500 mg. magnesium gluconate three times a day) may be required.

Zinc deficiency may cause the loss of the senses of smell and taste. Patients with these symptoms may benefit from supplementation with zinc sulfate (220 mg. three times a day).

SALT AND FLUID RESTRICTION. Cirrhosis disturbs the regulation of body salt and water. Severe liver disease generates neural and hormonal signals to the kidney that cause the kidney to retain both salt and water. The salt acts like a sponge. As a result, fluid accumulates in certain tissues and body spaces, such as the ankles (peripheral edema), abdomen (ascites), and chest (pleural effusion).

Treatment of fluid retention always requires dietary salt restriction, often requires diuretics (medicines that block the kidney and cause increased urination of salt and water), and sometimes requires fluid restriction. Patients need to understand that the major driving force behind the accumulation of fluid is the excessive retention of salt. Diuretics work because they cause the kidney to lose salt. If you take in too much salt in your diet, you'll cause more fluid to accumulate in your body. In other words, you can override the effects of the diuretics, and patients on diuretics can actually retain fluid if they don't comply with a salt-restricted diet.

The usual salt restriction is 2 grams per day. Commonly used diuretics are Aldactone (spironolactone), Midamor (amiloride), Lasix (furosemide), HCTZ (hydrochlorothiazide), and Zaroxylyn (metolozone). Aldactone and Midamor conserve potassium, while Lasix, HCTZ, and Zaroxylyn waste potassium. Most of the time, a doctor will prescribe the two types of diuretics together to minimize any changes in blood potassium levels. Occasionally, potassium supplements are used to keep blood potassium in the normal range.

The physician usually orders fluid restriction only for edematous (swollen with fluid) patients with low levels of sodium in their blood. Fluid restriction means restriction of all fluids: water, tea, coffee, milk, etc. Patients with severe symptomatic low blood sodium may find it necessary to restrict their fluid intake to less than 1 quart a day.

CAUTION: Always consult with your physician regarding use of diuretics (doses and frequency) or dietary restrictions on salt or fluid intake. It is potentially dangerous to self-medicate or introduce dietary restrictions without physician consultation.

> I'll make thee eat iron like an ostrich, and swallow my sword.
> WILLIAM SHAKESPEARE
> *King Henry VI*

REFERENCE
1. "Q and A's on Dietary Guidelines for Americans, 2000." 3 June 2000, *Center for Nutrition Policy and Promotion.* 1 Sept. 2000 , <www.usda.gov/cnpp/Pubs/DG2000/Qa5-2.pdf>.

7

TAKING CARE OF
YOURSELF EMOTIONALLY

Coping with a Genetic Condition

*I was devastated when I learned I had the double mutation. I passed
it on to my kids, but I didn't realize it wasn't my fault. I had never heard
of hemochromatosis.*

*It's like, "What did I do? Should I not have had kids?" Between my
two daughters getting me stuff off the Internet, I was so depressed the
first week or so that I was crying all the time.*

*My daughters said, "You couldn't know. It's not your fault. Thou-
sands of people have it and they don't know." It took me a couple of
weeks. Then I got over it.*

*What made me feel really bad is that my two grandchildren have
it—and they're only 8 to 10 years old.*

JILL

PEOPLE AFFECTED BY HEREDITARY HEMOCHRO-
matosis face a wide range of emotional challenges, depending
on the severity of their symptoms. If you have advanced
hemochromatosis, you must deal with serious chronic illness. If
you are fortunate enough to have been diagnosed early, before organ damage occurred, you still have to handle lifelong treatment issues. And, of
course, the hereditary nature of HH stirs up all kinds of family feelings.

Here are the topics we'll cover:

- **The Emotional Challenge**
- **Phase 1: Diagnosis**
  SPECIAL PROBLEMS WITH A DIAGNOSIS OF
  HEMOCHROMATOSIS
- **Phase 2: Impact (Attitudes and Expectations)**
- **Phase 3: Reorganization**
- **Healing vs. Curing**
- **Warning Signs of Depression**
- **Understanding your Family and Friends (Family Systems)**
  BOUNDARIES
- **Tools for Wellness: Some Practical Suggestions**
  MEDICAL CARE, PSYCHOLOGICAL HELP
    Genetic Counseling
    Information and Attitudes
    Support Groups
  EXERCISE AND NUTRITION
  FEELING USEFUL/HAVING FUN
  EXPLORING YOUR CREATIVE AND SPIRITUAL SIDES

The Emotional Challenge

A genetic condition, such as hemochromatosis, presents subtle and complex emotional challenges. You were born with a genetic time bomb. Nothing you did or didn't do contributed to your having the mutated genes of HH.

Why, then, do parents report a sense of guilt over passing hemochromatosis on to future generations? Why do some family members welcome information about genetic testing while others resent it? How do you deal with the anger and frustration of being misdiagnosed or diagnosed late? And if you were diagnosed too late to avoid organ damage and disease, how do you deal with chronic illness without letting it take over your life?

I would rather my son didn't have HH. But at the same time, my father didn't know he had it so he couldn't tell me. The difference is that I can help my son not end up like me, waiting for a liver transplant. I don't feel guilty, but I wish it were a different way. I'm not guilty over

*something that I had no control over, anymore than I blame my dad, and
I don't think my son blames me.*

*My dad would have done anything to help me—and I've been able
to help my son.*

GARY

"A genetic metabolic condition is no one's fault. Yet people, particularly parents, struggle with a sense of guilt, even though they themselves inherited hemochromatosis from their parents," says Meredith Pate-Willig, a licensed clinical social worker. Ms. Pate-Willig facilitates support groups for Denver's Qualife, an organization that seeks to enrich the quality of life for people facing life-challenging illness.

Annette K. Taylor, M.S., Ph.D., President and Laboratory Director of Kimball Genetics, cites one case where a woman's husband died after a prolonged, undiagnosed illness. On autopsy, the doctors found cirrhosis and increased iron stored in his liver. "The wife wanted an answer for her husband's death," says Taylor. "She was afraid her children or her husband's siblings might become sick and die, too."

The husband's DNA test result revealed two copies of the C282Y mutation, which is diagnostic of hemochromatosis. Taylor recommended that his siblings have DNA testing, because they each were at significant risk to have two copies of the same mutation (see Chapter 4). She also suggested that the children be tested.

"For the wife," says Taylor, " DNA testing of her husband was important. It helped bring closure to this situation and to identify other family members at risk."

"I don't know if we understand what the emotional impact of being identified with a genetic predisposition to a common, treatable disorder like hereditary hemochromatosis is going to be," says Carol Walton, M.S., C.G.C., Director of the Graduate Program in Genetic Counseling at the University of Colorado Health Sciences Center. "Traditionally, most disorders diagnosed genetically have been rare and largely untreatable. Clearly, people with HH may have to deal with chronic disease, which may potentially change their self-perception and does mean that they need to be on an ongoing medical regimen of treatment and monitoring. That, in and of itself, changes people's lives and whether they see themselves as sick or healthy individuals."

"To move on," says Pate-Willig, "You have to go through a grieving process about your changed sense of yourself. There's no shortcut through normal, natural cycles of grief. Grieving is nature's way of helping us adapt to new information about our illness."

Grieving is one way we work through loss. Sometimes it's loss of what we see as our old selves ("I never worried about my health before I found out I have hemochromatosis. Now if I go on a vacation, I have to make sure I'm near a place where I can get medical care."). Or it may be the loss of our dreams ("My mother was always so sick. Just before she died, we found out she had HH. I always thought she'd be a great grandma with my kids, but she never got the chance."). According to Pate-Willig, "Grieving is normal—even necessary. It's the bridge between what was to what is. If you don't go across that bridge, you may face a continuing struggle."

Too often, we're hard on ourselves as we grieve. In a world of instant cereal and microwave popcorn, we think we should be grieving faster, better. The truth is, each one of us goes through the process in our own time frame and in our own way—and the healing ingredient is kindness. Be patient with yourself. You will work it through, and you will come out of the crisis with a stronger sense of who you are.

According to Pate-Willig, it's helpful to think of these spiraling cycles of grief in three phases: diagnosis, impact, and reorganization.

Phase 1: Diagnosis

Diagnosis plunges you into a state of disbelief or shock. However, for people who have anxiously gone from doctor to doctor searching for a reason for their symptoms, diagnosis can bring a profound sense of relief as well.

> *My doctor, who's a caring, compassionate guy, said that they were told in medical school, "You'll never see a case of hemochromatosis because it's so rare. And if you do, it will be an older man."*
>
> *Half the battle is finding a doctor who takes you seriously and doesn't think it's all in your head.*
>
> SUSAN

In this first phase of diagnosis, you need your family and support system to pull together to help you adjust. Unfortunately, at the same time that you need support, your family members are trying to deal with anxiety about their own tests for HH. In addition, you may feel doubly anxious about the test results of your spouse or children.

- *A diagnosis of hereditary hemochromatosis may make you uncomfortable or leave you with a numbing sense of shock and loss. You should understand that these responses are normal.*
- *Everyone needs psychological and social support—not just the person diagnosed with hemochromatosis. When one part of a system changes, everything in the system reacts in a "ripple" effect.*
- *People who have lost family members to hemochromatosis might have a stronger reaction to the diagnosis than people who have family members who were diagnosed early and are doing quite well.*
- *The diagnosis raises questions about family relationships. Who else in your family has HH? Whom should you alert? Why does John seem grateful for the information while Laura refuses to talk about it?*

People may not respond to you in the way that you anticipate or expect. You may process the information fast while family members take longer, or the reverse. How fast or how slowly people absorb the news affects the dynamics in a marriage or friendship—leaving everyone with the unconscious feeling that somehow the rules changed. In fact, just identifying these changes takes a while.

> *My mother is the oldest of 15 children. I wrote to them all. To this day I have tried to explain that she and my father had to be at least carriers. I actually think my father had full-blown HH, because I ache in the same places he did.*
>
> *I didn't get any response from my relatives. I guess they thought, "She's got it. So what does that have to do with me?"*
>
> *HH goes from one generation to another. It bothers me that my brother and sister don't get tested, and their kids haven't been tested*
>
> ESTHER

Sometimes, the patient or support system refuses to accept the new reality. "Denial," says Pate-Willig, "is a misunderstood defense. When it acts as a circuit-breaker, it keeps your system from overloading. That can be healthy. Denial becomes unhealthy when it keeps you from finding appropriate medical treatment."

SPECIAL PROBLEMS WITH A DIAGNOSIS OF HEMOCHROMATOSIS. Dealing with a diagnosis of any chronic condition is difficult, but patients with hemochromatosis have special issues:

Feeling Low. You may be experiencing fatigue, low energy, and a reduced ability to do your daily tasks. These "silent" symptoms may make you more emotionally vulnerable and susceptible to periods of depression. Be sure to tell your doctor if you feel seriously depressed.

> *I was working as a camp counselor when my energy level dropped. I had always been anemic so I started eating iron-rich foods like spinach and beef. I took iron pills—the whole nine yards.*
>
> *In the fall, I was still exhausted. I slept a lot. I'm a great believer in your body telling you what's wrong so I got my blood tested. My ferritin was 275. My doctor wasn't concerned. "You'll never be anemic," he said.*
>
> *But my mother is a nurse, and we looked up ferritin in a 1972 Merck manual. Right there it talked about hemochromatosis and said that normal ferritin ranges are from 10 to 65.*
>
> ELISE

Looking Good. If you are in the early stages of HH, you probably don't look sick. If your skin is bronzed from HH, you may even appear healthily suntanned.

> *I spent a year working in Hawaii. I tanned from head to toe. After two years, I couldn't figure out why I didn't lose the tan. It was bronzing.*
>
> KEN

Unfortunately, many people (including yourself) may have a hard time believing that you are dealing with some difficult issues. Unless you explain the nature of hemochromatosis, you may not get the support you need.

Sense of Isolation. Although hemochromatosis is a common genetic condition, most people have never heard of it. HH doesn't get much press. When you confide in others, you may get blank looks at first, and you'll have to educate your family and friends.

> *It's isolating. I don't know people with HH. Once I met a guy at the blood bank. Mostly I read about it on the Internet, but they don't update the pages much.*
>
> FRANK

Frustration with Delayed Diagnosis. Doctors confuse symptoms of HH with diseases or conditions such as alcoholism, arthritis, or impotence. In some cases, doctors have referred patients to psychiatrists without diagnosing the underlying physical problem. A 1996–1997 survey, supported by the Centers for Disease Control and Prevention, involved a questionnaire sent to 3,562 HH patients. Of the 2,851 HH patients who responded, 67 percent had been diagnosed with an alternate condition. People with symptoms were diagnosed with hemochromatosis only after the symptoms had been present, on average, for 10 years and after visiting an average of 3.5 physicians.

> *I first began to realize I was having a problem with my liver when I started retaining fluids. The doctors assumed it was alcohol, so I ran around with that situation for a couple of months.*
> *But I'm not an alcoholic. I wasn't tested for HH until I was on the liver transplant list!*
>
> SAUL

Misdiagnosis leads to frustration, anger, fear, uncertainty, and a feeling of helplessness. If permanent organ damage has occurred because of a delayed diagnosis, these feelings are heightened.

Genetic Information Overload. The field of genetics is exploding with information. Even experts have difficulty keeping up. It's easy to feel overwhelmed when you are trying to understand how a genetic condition like HH can affect your life (see the section on Genetic Counseling, Chapter 3).

This genetic stuff is hard to understand. When I first heard the words homozygous and heterozygous, I didn't know what they were talking about at all.

GINA

Uncertainty. As with all genetic conditions, there is no way to predict the exact course of hemochromatosis in any one individual. That's because we are all unique. Many factors influence our health, such as the environment, alcohol consumption, other illnesses, and so on.

At our family reunion, I was so bloated that the bottoms of my feet were rounded. I just waddled. And I heard one cousin whisper, "I don't think she'll be here next year."

WILLA

Family Factors. Because HH is a family condition, the discovery of HH in one person means that others have to be notified. Even when the family is close and connected, this is an anxious time—although it's also an opportunity to strengthen ties. However, if communication problems already exist (and what family doesn't have some issues), stress increases.

I'm a bachelor with no siblings. My mom blamed herself for giving me hemochromatosis. I wrote a four-page letter to my family telling them about HH—first cousins, aunts, etc., and I got a 90 percent response rate. People got tested. They sent me newspaper clippings.

But one branch of the family never wrote back. My mother said, "They probably blame you. We're the black sheep of the family now."

Bam! That Christmas we got no card from anyone in that branch of the family—and we had been getting cards since 1920.

RALPH

Family structures run the gamut from families that don't want to know anything to families that push members to absorb the information—even when they don't want to. Who becomes the gatekeeper of information? Whom are we obligated to tell and why? Do we tell in person or write a letter? How much do we tell?

Genetic Discrimination. Genetic advances are racing ahead of the legal and ethical questions that they raise. Will your diagnosis of HH affect your job opportunities or your health and insurance coverage? We hope you will never suffer discrimination, but the threat is omnipresent. (For information about genetic discrimination, see Chapter 8.)

What Can You Do to Help Yourself? "Be patient with yourself," says Pate-Willig. "Accept that this is a difficult time, and try not to beat yourself up for being normal, human."

"Remember to be kind to yourself. Patience, patience, and more patience. That's the key," says Pate-Willig. "Expect to feel emotional cycles, ups and downs, each time the activity of your disease changes or you experience a new symptom."

Phase 2: Impact (Attitudes and Expectations)

In Phase 1, the task for you and your support system is to pull together to understand the new diagnosis. In the second phase, the question becomes, "How do we function now that we know that hemochromatosis is a lifelong condition? How do we gear up for the long haul?" It's a time of changing attitudes and expectations as you explore your options.

The challenge is how to connect with friends and family and still maintain the autonomy and space you need. Your questions may vary from "How much help can I ask from my family now that I need a liver transplant?" to "My wife nags me about maintenance phlebotomies. How do I tell her nicely to back off?"

Families often have unspoken rules and myths about illness. Perhaps the message you got was, "Keep a stiff upper lip and don't show you're scared." Or maybe you grew up in a home where a cold meant you got to stay in bed all day. What happens if you break these rules?

> I have a large family—five older brothers, a sister, and twenty-two nieces and nephews. I told my family to take the genetic test and find out if they were prone to develop HH. Some didn't even do that. It's something that people don't like to address.
>
> One older brother and one nephew have been diagnosed. I just hope my nephew is getting proper treatment.
>
> I went to a funeral and was in the car with four of my family. I asked if anyone took the gene test. No one said, "Thanks for alerting me. I really appreciate it."

My brother died of liver cancer, but his kids didn't seem concerned for themselves. It's their life to live. All I can do is alert them—and go on with my life.

ERIC

"The discovery of a genetic disease in a family can potentially impact a family's ability to communicate," says Walton. "This is based on feelings of blame ("I have this disorder because you gave it to me"), guilt for passing on the disorder ("How could my child inherit this from me when I am a healthy person?"), or even survivor guilt ("My sibling has this, and I don't. I feel bad that my sibling is going through this."). "But," cautions Walton, "Our understanding of these reactions in adults is largely based on disorders such as Huntington's disease and hereditary cancer syndromes."

Sharing genetic information can have an unexpected impact on family communication. One study conducted in the Netherlands involved eighteen people at risk for Huntington's disease a year after testing. After the initial shock (Huntington's disease is hereditary and can lead to death), the nine people with the faulty gene for Huntington's seemed to cope well with the unfavorable test results.

The unexpected finding concerned the people who did not carry the faulty gene. Although not one of these people regretted having the test, eight reported that their initial relief was replaced by guilt and depression. Six avoided contact with siblings; family members seemed indifferent to their test results. Two did not tell their siblings what the results were. Four reported that relatives reacted by "banning" them from the family. In other words, the genetic threat had created a bond for family members.

The authors of the study discussed reasons why those who did not carry the faulty gene may have found it difficult to deal with survivor's guilt. Why did they escape the disease? Perhaps they felt that because they did not inherit the genes, they put their siblings more at risk. In addition, there may have been a feeling of obligation to be more supportive and available to at-risk members. Spouses of the at-risk members needed support also, but may have found their needs overshadowed by the attention focused on the affected person.

What do we know about the emotional effects of a diagnosis of HH? The CDC-supported survey questionnaire, published in 1999, asked people with HH about changes in their lives (Table 7). Not surprisingly,

60 percent of those who did not have severe hemochromatosis reported no real life change. In contrast, 71 percent of people with severe HH reported that the diagnosis changed their life significantly. (Severe HH was defined as a diagnosis of disease due to HH, such as diabetes, arthritis, liver disease, etc., or self-reported skin bronzing.) This difference indicates that chronic illness due to HH, rather than HH alone, significantly impacts a person's life.

Not all changes were negative. For example, some people reported divorces while others said their marriages grew stronger. An interesting finding was that a greater percentage of family members of patients who had severe HH were in denial of the patient's disease or in denial of their own risk.

TABLE 7 : LIFE CHANGES REPORTED BY PATIENTS WITH HEMOCHRO-
MATOSIS, BY SEVERITY OF HEMOCHROMATOSIS*[1]

TYPE OF CHANGE	WITH SEVERE HEMO-CHROMATOSIS (N=1255)	WITHOUT SEVERE HEMO-CHROMATOSIS (N=1596)
	% REPORTING	% REPORTING
DIVORCE OR BREAKUP WITH SIGNIFICANT OTHER	6.5	2.0
TROUBLES WITH SPOUSE OR SIGNIFICANT OTHER	7.7	1.4
MARRIAGE OR RELATIONSHIP STRONGER	13.4	4.8
FAMILY MEMBERS IN DENIAL OF MY DISEASE	12.3	3.8
FAMILY MEMBERS IN DENIAL OF OWN RISK	25.2	12.7
FAMILY MEMBERS SUPPORTIVE	44.5	38.1
JOB LOSS	19.6	2.8
REDUCED ABILITY TO DO DAILY TASKS	33.4	7.3
LOSS OF HEALTH INSURANCE	8.7	5.8
LOSS OF LIFE INSURANCE	7.7	6.4
OTHER	5.6	3.3
NO REAL CHANGE	28.7	60.0

*Severe hemochromatosis = physician diagnosis of either liver disease (including cirrhosis), diabetes mellitus, hypothyroidism, hypogonadism, or arthritis, or joint replacement, liver transplant, or self-reported skin bronzing.

Phase 3: Reorganization

As you move into Phase 3, you and your family begin to reorganize around the new reality. A sense of acceptance emerges, and you start to answer these questions: Who am I now? How am I going to make my life work?

> *I time my maintenance phlebotomies to fit my work schedule. I have to go every three months, and I teach—so I do them on my school breaks.*
>
> *Before, HH took over my life and controlled me. Now I feel I have control over it. Now phlebotomies and blood tests are just a part of my life.*
>
> JULIANA

At some point, things settle down. Perhaps you come to terms with a reduced energy level, make dietary changes, decide on a treatment plan.

Anything that tips the precarious balancing act shakes the system. If you start phlebotomy treatment and it tires you out, you and your family and friends may need to organize around the treatment. Suppose you decide to plan a nap each day, while someone else assumes your chores. What most people don't realize is that any change, positive or negative, alters the system. So, paradoxically, you may need to reorganize when you switch to less frequent maintenance treatments. For example, you may still feel the need for a daily nap, but the people around you may now disapprove.

The cycle of confronting the diagnosis, feeling its impact, and reorganizing to deal with hemochromatosis may recur with each piece of health news. If HH moves into advanced liver disease and a possible transplant, the concept of death may come to the forefront.

"The first big breakthrough for most people is the realization of how physically fragile we humans are," says Pate-Willig. "It's a difficult task to process, reprioritize, accept your mortality, and—at the same time—plan for post-transplant living."

Healing vs. Curing

"We are all desperate for curing," says Pate-Willig, "but a physical cure may be years away. We need to shift to healing—a balance and wholeness of mind, body, and spirit.

"As we become more aware of our emotional responses, we learn how healthy it is to lean into the grief process and accept it. We learn how to tap into resources that can help, such as dietary changes and relaxation techniques. The goal is to come out of each cycle at a higher level, to feel better about ourselves, and to see more flexibility in ourselves and others as we learn how to cope."

Grief can be the great healer. Grief is to the psyche and the spirit what the physical process is to the healing of a wound. But how does one find an outlet for grief?

"Talk about what's happening to you," says Pate-Willig. Talk to a friend, a support group. Keep a journal. Get on the Internet. Help yourself by reevaluating your feelings each time you tell and retell your story. As you do this, you fit your new self into your old idea of yourself.

> *When I first found out I had hemochromatosis, it was overwhelming, scary. Talking to other people who have it makes me feel not so alone. It brings comfort.*
>
> TERRIE

"The Chinese symbol for crisis is both danger and opportunity. Chronic illness can give us the opportunity to become deeper, broader, more flexible, and to find meaning in our lives."

Warning Signs of Depression

While grieving and depression are normal, sustained depression is not. Fortunately, there are many ways to treat depression with medications and "talk" therapy, so it's important to tell your doctor, advises Robert House, M.D., Director of Residency Training and the Department of Psychiatric Consultation Liason Service for the University of Colorado Health Sciences Center.

What are the signs of depression? According to Dr. House, be on the alert for some of these symptoms, if they are changes from your normal behavior pattern:

- *Low energy, fatigue, lack of interest in your usual activities*
- *Withdrawn and/or irritable behavior*
- *Sleep disturbances that show a change in your routine pattern (such as sleeping less or more, waking up a lot, or waking earlier or later than usual, not rested and ready to begin the day)*

- *Significant weight loss over a short period of time*
- *Loss of appetite, food doesn't taste good*
- *Tearfulness, breaking into tears for no apparent reason, "out of the blue"*
- *Forming and talking about ideas of suicide, or a sense that life is not worth living*
- *Feeling hopeless, helpless, that things won't get better*
- *Reluctance to resume activities of daily living after a medical procedure such as a transplant (examples: not getting along with your family, if you've always done so before; not resuming sexual relations with your spouse after a reasonable length of time; not dating, if single; isolating yourself from others).*

RESOURCE: For more information on depression, contact the National Institute of Mental Health (NIMH) Public Inquiries, 6001 Executive Boulevard, Room 8184, MSC 9663, Bethesda, MD 20892-9663. Phone: 301-443-4513; Fax: 301-443-4279; TTY: 301-443-8431. Ask for a pamphlet titled "Depression," NIH No. 00-3561, or access the NIH Web site: www.nimh.nih.gov/publicat/depression.cfm. In addition, the following Web sites are helpful: Health Topics at www.medlineplus.gov; National Mental Health Association at www.nmha.org.

Understanding Your Family and Friends (Family Systems)

I got the double whammy of my parents, but my brothers and sisters didn't have any mutated genes. I felt all alone.

After I sent an alarming letter to all my extended relatives, I felt kind of dumb, because I'm the only one with HH.

Some relatives resented the cost of testing. One guy blamed me because everyone in his family turned out negative. You'd think when they were warned, they'd be happy. But telling your relatives is something you need to do. If they don't take it well, it's their problem.

My little brother created a family website. He posted the information about my HH so that when family members go for blood work or physicals, they'll test for iron.

Chronic illness is a family illness—especially when it is a genetic condition. When one member of a family becomes sick, it affects everyone. Normally, a family stays in balance with its own set of unwritten roles and rules. Roles involve position (Who is the breadwinner? Who takes out the garbage?). Roles always change as the patient needs to do less and shifts tasks to others. Rules are values; they can be about communication (Who is the gatekeeper about HH information?), emotion (Who is allowed to be sad?), education, sex, religion, and parenting.

Most important for people with more advanced hemochromatosis are the family rules and values about health and illness. Problems arise when your family rules (or the rules of the family you grew up in) clash. Can you take time off if you have a cold or only if you're deathly ill? How do you handle the medical system?

BOUNDARIES. Families create different boundaries. Some are so enmeshed that it's hard to tell where one member begins and another ends. They know how to pull together but need to learn how to allow outsiders to help. At the other end of the spectrum is the disengaged family in which members have a high degree of autonomy and very little meaningful communication with each other. They need to learn how to draw closer, so they can hear each other and support one another. Most families, of course, fall somewhere between these two extremes.

Chronic illness can cause disorganization, but this crisis can open more options and choices as the family modifies and changes its rules and values.

Families also go through life stages that have their own issues of separateness and connectedness, from the birth of a child to taking care of elderly parents. When illness occurs, it can disrupt the normal tasks of these life stages. Suppose, for example, that severe hemochromatosis with, for example, cirrhosis or liver cancer strikes a parent of a teenager. The teenager will feel pulled by conflicting forces: the need to separate and develop a life with peers versus the need to pull closer to the family. In this setting the adolescent must cope with developing separateness and freedom and providing more help with household or other chores.

Communication and openness are the keys to improving the level of understanding within your family. When family members talk about a problem in terms of shifts in roles, rules and life stages, it diffuses the personal element. Usually, people feel hurt when a conflict arises because they think the other family members don't care about them. When you

define the problem as a conflict in family roles, values, or degree of sep-
aration/connection, you can work toward a resolution.

Suppose, for example, that George wants his wife, Susan, to drive him
to all his medical appointments at the liver transplant center. Meanwhile,
Susan has had to take a part-time job to help pay the bills. Even though
it's no one's fault, she's angry. Susan can't do it all. Her former role as the
family's primary emotional support needs to be modified. Instead of
blaming each other and feeling unloved, Susan and George talk about
the role changes and come up with a compromise. Susan will go to the
important medical appointments, and George will ask his sister to
accompany him to the routine ones.

Do people want to change a family system? No, but illness brings
unavoidable changes and, therefore, a feeling of loss of control. You can
choose to be angry or you can decide what can be changed and what
cannot. How can we figure out a new system that's fair to everybody?
What roles and values can we let go or modify?

Tools for Wellness: Some Practical Suggestions

Life-challenging illnesses, such as severe and advanced hemochromatosis, present opportunities for rethinking priorities. We may not always be
able to cure the disease, but we can improve the quality of our lives. We
can nourish ourselves by getting good medical and psychological care,
exercising, eating nutritious foods, trying to live meaningful and useful
lives, deepening relationships, having fun, and exploring our creative and
spiritual sides.

Adapt an open and curious attitude when exploring these areas, and
don't try all of them at once. Make changes gradually. Here are some
suggestions from Pate-Willig and others:

CAUTION: Specific recommendations regarding diet, nutrition,
and exercise may vary and should be evaluated and discussed with your
physician.

MEDICAL CARE, PSYCHOLOGICAL HELP. Put together your medical
team with care. The treatment of hemachromatosis requires knowledge
of specialized tests and treatments. Many doctors don't have much experience with HH, so find a gastroenterologist, hepatologist, or hematologist who does. Most medical centers have specialists or can recommend
appropriate community specialists.

If your doctor's standard answer is that everything checks out okay, but you know it's not okay, you have to be your own advocate. If your doctor can't find the answer, you need to find another doctor.

My family doctor is my hero. I laud him and honor him for his quick diagnosis.

You have to empower yourself with as much knowledge as possible. And you have to manage your health. I find I have to be assertive with my doctor. I say things like, "I need you to help me understand this. I need you to be here with me right now. I have to write this down.

When my former doctor wanted to dismiss me, I started keeping my own records. I always ask for copies of my reports and tests. As you get older, things kind of slip. This way I can go back and check facts. My lab papers and reports alone are an inch thick. My notebook, which I've kept since 1992, measures 1 1/2 inches.

Although credentials are important, effective therapy may also be dependent upon the doctor-patient relationship. Make sure that the two of you are a good fit. This is a very individual matter. Do you like your doctor to tell you exactly what to do, or do you prefer to have more input with decision-making? Does the doctor answer your questions fully, or seem eager to exit? Do the nurses and receptionist seem friendly and supportive?

RESOURCE: Many of the national organizations listed in Resources at the end of this book, such as the American Hemochromatosis Society and others, can refer you to centers and physicians in your area who specialize in hemochromatosis.

RESOURCE: Access the GeneTests-GeneClinics Web site to search for the genetic clinic nearest you. The government-funded site is free, but you will be asked to register. Web site: www.geneclinics.org

Genetic Counseling. Genetic counselors help people understand their condition and facilitate decision-making about medical management and genetic issues. Many physicians specializing in genetic disorders, geneticists (board-certified physicians), and genetic counselors provide genetic counseling. A genetics counselor should have a degree in genetic counseling from an accredited master's level graduate program. Check to see if the counselor is board certified by the American Board of Genetic Counseling (ABGC). If you live in a rural area, ask the nearest academic medical center if they provide outreach clinics. (See Chapter 3, Genetic Tests, for more information on genetic counseling.)

A genetics counselor typically does not provide long-term therapy. If you need to see a mental health professional (psychologist, psychiatrist, social worker, professional counselor), your genetics counselor can refer you or you can get names from friends you trust and interview a few practitioners. Ask about their backgrounds and qualifications. Make sure they have experience in dealing with issues of chronic illness. They should be graduates of an accredited master's or Ph.D. program and licensed by the state as an independent practitioner or supervised by someone who is licensed.

RESOURCE: The National Society of Genetic Counselors, Inc. (NSGC) features a "ResourceLink" on its Web site that lists genetic counselors by state, city, and specialty. The NSGC is located at 233 Canterbury Dr., Wallingford, PA 19086. Phone: 610-872-7608; Web site: www.nsgc.org

RESOURCE: Tagliaferro, Linda and Mark V. Bloom, Ph.D. *The Complete Idiot's Guide to Decoding Your Genes.* New York: Alpha Books/Macmillan, 1999.

Information and Attitudes. Keep abreast of developments in HH research. The more you know, the better your decisions will be. (See Chapter 12, Research Trends. Consider joining some of the organizations listed in the Resources section at the back of this book to receive newsletters that will keep you up to date.)

Finally, look at your own beliefs and attitudes about illness. Learn what works for you and what doesn't. We don't choose to be sick, but we can choose how we try to handle the situation.

RESOURCES ON HEMOCHROMATOSIS:
Crawford, Roberta. *tick...tick...tick....* Glyndon: Vida, 1994. (a medical mystery novel involving HH)
Crawford, Roberta. *The Iron Elephant.* 2nd ed. Glyndon: Vida, 2000. (HH information)
Iron Disorders Institute. *Guide to Hemochromatosis.* Nashville: Cumberland House, 2001. (HH information)
Kane, Terry. *Sick in America.* Denver: Silverman Press, 1996. (autobiographical account of one man's journey with HH)
Warder, Marie. *The Bronze Killer.* Delta: Imperani, 1999. (autobiographical story of a family's fight against hemochromatosis by the founder of several HH associations, including the Canadian Hemochromatosis Society)
GENERAL RESOURCES:
Bridges, William. *Transitions.* Reading: Addison-Wesley, 1980.

Clarke, Peter & Susan H. Evans. *Surviving Modern Medicine, How to Get the Best from Doctors, Family & Friends.* New Brunswick: Rutgers University Press, 1998.

Flach, Frederic, M.D. *Resilience: The Power to Bounce Back When the Going Gets Tough.* New York: Hatherleigh Press, 1997.

Kushner, Harold S. *When Bad Things Happen to Good People.* New York: Avon, 1981.

Travis, John W., M.D. and Regina Sara Ryan. *Wellness Workbook.* Berkeley: Ten Speed Press, 1988.

Support Groups. Many studies prove the importance of support systems. The results of one well-known study, reported in 1989 by psychiatrist David Spiegel and colleagues, showed that women with metastatic breast cancer who attended weekly group therapy sessions lived significantly longer than those who did not.[2]

Most of us benefit from a network of informal supportive relationships. Effective support always includes a sharing of emotions and feelings—a quality of reciprocity. Each person feels heard, validated, and has a sense of being able to draw upon that support, if necessary.

One man who came to our support group was so bronze-colored that we just gasped. And he sounded so tired.

Support groups are important because we know what it's like to go through this. You have to have support somewhere to know that you are not alone. My doctor told me HH is very rare. Then we learn that it's the most common genetic disorder. How many people out there have it and are without a clue? Or are tired, like me, and the doctor says to take iron pills?

When I found out I had hemochromatosis, I jumped on the Internet. I found a couple of societies of people who had HH. A lot of them were people who'd had an experience like mine—being called an alcoholic even though they never drank.

Our support group has a sense of humor. Sometimes we're confused and forgetful and get "brain fog" from iron overload. So we made up a new word for ourselves using Fe, the symbol for iron. We call ourselves "Fe-brains."

I haven't missed a single meeting of my support group, even when the weather is bad. I learn information when the doctors come and show slides. I learn from other people in the group, and I think my sharing is helpful to them.

With any of these medical problems, knowledge helps. You have a better chance of being able to do something if you don't do the ostrich thing.

I'm the only one in my support group who admits to erectile dysfunction and talks about it. Some people think it's an admission of weakness. Be a man! I like to share the information so people can be helped.

I just joined a support group on Yahoo.com. You have to register, pick a name, a password. For me, the Internet is good, because I live in a rural area. There are twenty to thirty posts a day so I go on every day, or they pile up. I weed them out. Only a few people say something worthwhile, and you get to know which posts to read after a while. Most people just put down doctors, and I get tired of reading that.

My support group is wonderful. People listen. 'This is what happened to me. I have been there, too. This is how I handled it.' We take the information and adapt it to our own situations.

Formal support groups are useful because they provide a common experience for patients, a sense of not being alone, and a safe place to share feelings and information.

"People feel so alone, so isolated," says Sandra Thomas, President and founder of the American Hemochromatosis Society. "Sometimes you feel that you are the only person in the world who has this condition. But in this computer age we can reach out and support each other with online discussion groups. There were only five people in our first support group. Now, our listserv, Families HHelping Families, has approximately 500 people!"

RESOURCE: Contact the American Hemochromatosis Society for information about its online support group (Families HHelping Families Circle). Phone: 1-888-655-IRON (4766)—a 24-hour toll-free information hotline Web site: www.americanhs.org Email: mail@americanhs.org

RESOURCE: The Genetic Alliance offers a free genetics Helpline staffed by genetic counselors, Mon.–Fri., 9:00AM to 5:00PM EST. Phone: 1-800-336-GENE. Email: info@geneticalliance.org

RESOURCE: If you'd like to start your own HH support group, the Genetic Alliance has a helpful packet titled "The Making of a Self-Help Group" for a $2 handling charge. You may order via their online publication order form or write to Genetic Alliance, 4301 Connecticut Ave., NW #404, Washington, DC 20008-2304. Website: www.geneticalliance.org

EXERCISE AND NUTRITION. Physical movement not only strengthens your body, it helps your emotional state. If you can afford it, a personal trainer with experience in chronic illness is helpful. Hospitals often have cardiac or stroke rehabilitation experts who may be able to refer you to the right professional, but you don't need money to exercise. You can walk with a friend, rent yoga or tai chi videos, or try water exercise to avoid stress on painful joints. Be creative.

I run a mile a day, do Pilates, walk, and rollerblade. Oh yes, I also do endurance horseracing. I eat a low carbohydrate diet, but when I'm doing a lot of outdoor exercising, I increase the carbs.

Through all the arthritis, I kept working out at a fitness club. I think it's a real factor in recovery. I try to take two classes a week. I attend a one-hour stretch class, and then I work on selected variable weight machines. I'm trying to maintain my strength, build it if I can, and maintain as good a range of motion as I can—and I'm in my seventies.

Also, it's a wonderful social support system. I've been going for fourteen years. I've made a lot of friends there. We have a great time together.

For information on nutrition, see Chapter 6, Taking Care of Yourself Nutritionally.

CAUTION: Consult your doctor before you begin any exercise program or make dietary changes.

FEELING USEFUL/HAVING FUN. We need a sense of meaning and purpose in our lives. We also need to have fun and play. Look for activities that create joy, hope, and a sense of living fully.

My wife gave me a Harley-Davidson. It's a little hard to shift gears and pull the clutch because it hurts my hand. Arthritis is probably the worst pain I've got.

I limp some in the mornings, and then it loosens up. But I've always been an active, healthy guy, and it pisses me off if there's something I can't do. So I ride my Harley.

I knew I was diagnosed in time, and that if HH was treated properly, it was not serious. I sent a letter to my family and selected friends to inform them and I decided to have a bit of fun with expressions about iron. For example, I wrote, "Already, my personality is more magnetic."

I have an engineer friend who works with metals, and he drafted a response using metallurgical terminology. He started the letter with "O Ferrous Friend."

I have a twin sister who has high iron levels. Women don't have problems until later in life, after the menstrual cycle ends, so she didn't have a buildup like me for a long, long time. She gets her blood checked and has phlebotomies once in a while.

You have to look for the positive, the meaning. My situation helped save her.

Ask yourself these questions: What is important to me? How am I acting on the important things in my life? How can I continue to have a meaningful existence within the limits of my health and energy levels?

RESOURCES:

Anderson, Greg. *50 Essential Things to Do When the Doctor Says It's Cancer.* New York: Penguin, 1993.

LeShan, Lawrence. *Cancer As a Turning Point.* New York: Penguin, 1994.

Topf, Linda Noble with Hal Z. Bennett. *You Are Not Your Illness.* New York: Fireside, 1995.

Playing helps you recapture joy. "Like humor, a good joyful experience does as much for your sense of well-being as a good physical workout," says Pate-Willig. It requires flexibility and a commitment to explore options. If you can't climb mountains anymore, investigate handicapped-accessible trails or rent travel videos. Open yourself to new experiences. If you've never explored poetry, for example, now may be the time to visit your neighborhood library.

"Learn to live mindfully," says Pate-Willig. "Ask yourself: 'Do I notice the people chattering at my dinner table, and am I grateful for my family? Do I savor the vivid colors of the vegetables I'm cutting? Do I stop for a moment during the day to notice that I feel good?'"

EXPLORING YOUR CREATIVE AND SPIRITUAL SIDES. Using the mind's capacity for healing includes visualization, relaxation, guided imagery, meditation, journal writing, and creative arts. All of these are ways to help the mind create a quieter atmosphere and to improve your quality of life.

Visualization, meditation, and relaxation create a sense of relaxed alertness and counteract the stress of daily living. Visit a bookstore and look over the tapes and videos. There are more than 30 methods, so the important thing is to find what makes you feel comfortable.

RESOURCES:

Benson, Herbert and Miriam Klipper. *The Relaxation Response.* New York: Avon, 1976.

Kabat-Zinn, Jon. Full Catastrophe Living. New York: Dell, 1990.

Journal writing lowers stress levels and can be your best friend in the middle of the night when there's no one else to talk to. Write quickly, don't censor yourself, and find a safe place to keep your journal.

RESOURCES:

Capacchione, Lucia. *The Well-Being Journal.* North Hollywood: Newcastle, 1989.

Remen, Rachel Naomi, M.D. *Kitchen Table Wisdom, Stories That Heal.* New York: Riverhead Books, 1996.

Creative art forms (painting, drawing, music, dance, poetry) are healing because you work with symbols and images to express feelings.

RESOURCE: Capacchione, Lucia. *The Creative Journal.* North Hollywood: Newcastle, 1989.

Guided imagery is a specific kind of relaxation and movement using the mind's own images. Most mental health professionals who deal with illness can assist you in creating an individual tape that works for you. A prerequisite is to practice relaxation so you can access guided imagery. The technique uses all five senses and works best when it's tailored to you. Not everyone sees images, for example. If that's the case with you, the therapist will use sounds or smells instead.

Even if you don't hold formal religious beliefs, you can tap into your spirituality, says Pate-Willig. "Think back to your feelings at the birth of your child, or when you suddenly came upon a bed of glorious wildflowers. Spirituality connects you with a sense of something larger than the self."

Illness, however, can also present a theological challenge. According to Dr. House, some patients "go through a crisis of faith. People who've gone to church all their lives may suddenly feel rejected, alone and abandoned, angry with God, or feel this illness is punishment for some unknown sin. Their social network is centered on their church, so if they lose this, they lose a lot. I recommend that they talk to their clergy or to the hospital chaplain."

"Spiritual distress," says Rev. Julie Swaney, Chaplain at the University of Colorado Health Sciences Center, "occurs when a person's faith or spirit is suddenly full of holes. Everything you believe in is gone. You've lost your value system, and you feel alone. But one of the gifts of illness is the way it opens us up to life. People reassess relationships, values, their sense of time, of what's important. Spirituality has to do with how we make meaning out of our experiences. Embrace what works for you."

RESOURCES:

Benson, Herbert, M.D., with Marg Stark. *Timeless Healing, The Power and Biology of Belief.* New York: Scribner, 1996.

Byock, Ira, M.D. *Dying Well, Peace and Possibilities at the End of Life.* New York: Riverhead Books, 1997.

Frankl, Victor E. *Man's Search for Meaning.* New York: Simon & Schuster, 1984.

Kushner, Harold S. *When All You've Ever Wanted Isn't Enough.* New York: Simon & Schuster, 1986.

Finally, one last word on being good to yourself: Take small steps to wellness slowly, over time. There is no correct formula. Make changes slowly so that you can keep your life in balance.

> *Nor airless dungeon, nor strong links of iron,*
> *Can be retentive to the strength of spirit.*
> WILLIAM SHAKESPEARE
> *Julius Caesar*

REFERENCES

1. Sharon M. McDonnell, MD, MPH, Ben L. Preston, BS, Sandy A. Jewell, MS, MPA, James C. Baron, MD, Corwin Q. Edwards, MD, Paul C. Adams, MD, Ray Yip, MD, MPH. "A Survey of 2,851 Patients with Hemochromatosis: Symptoms and Response to Treatment." *American Journal of Medicine* 106 (1999): 622.

2. David Spiegel, M.D. *Living Beyond Limits.* (New York: Random House, 1993), 79.

8

FINANCIAL IMPACT OF HEMOCHROMATOSIS

Treatment Costs and Insurance Factors

In 1996, I applied for a life insurance policy. The company did a liver function test, and my enzyme levels were on the high end of the scale. My family doctor said the numbers were barely out of the range of normal and not to worry about it. The policy was approved.

Last year, I reapplied for low rates, and my liver enzymes were so high they were off the map. I went to a different doctor who tested me. I had the C282Y mutation, both sides. "You're a slam dunk for hemochromatosis," he said.

With phlebotomies, I've gotten my enzyme levels down to normal. My headaches have stopped. My hair stopped thinning.

The company couldn't take away my life insurance policy, but I didn't qualify for cheaper rates. Today, I wouldn't be able to get a policy.

JEREMY

Y OU MAY FEEL TOO FATIGUED TO WORK, BUT you can't quit your job because you need to hold on to your health insurance. Perhaps the medical bills are piling up, and you're worried about paying the mortgage. Any chronic illness can put a dent in your budget.

Each one of you, however, faces a different situation. This chapter presents a general overview of financial issues, some helpful resources, and a discussion of genetic discrimination.*

We'll cover:

- ◆ **Cost of Treatment**
      PHLEBOTOMY COSTS
      CHELATION COSTS
      ONGOING MEDICAL CARE COSTS

- ◆ *Private Health Insurance*
      SELECTING HEALTH INSURANCE
      TYPES OF PRIVATE HEALTH INSURANCE: MANAGED CARE OR
      FEE-FOR-SERVICE
         HMOs
         PPOs
         Fee-for-Service Plans

- ◆ *Government Health Insurance*
      MEDICARE
      MEDICAID
      VETERANS ADMINISTRATION (VA)

- ◆ *When You're Too Sick to Work: Applying for Disability*
      SHORT-TERM DISABILITY LEAVE

- ◆ *Disability Insurance Resources*
      SOCIAL SECURITY DISABILITY INSURANCE (SSDI)
      SUPPLEMENTAL SECURITY INCOME (SSI)

- ◆ *Genetic Discrimination in Insurance and Employment*
      ARE THERE SAFEGUARDS AGAINST GENETIC
      DISCRIMINATION?

*NOTE: This chapter is an overview, not an exhaustive treatment of financial options and programs. It does not provide legal advice; always contact agencies and companies for specific information and consult a lawyer for legal advice in specific cases.

Cost of Treatment

PHLEBOTOMY COSTS. Your costs for phlebotomy therapy depend upon the number of treatments and where you are treated. A survey of phlebotomy practices, published in 1999, reported that of the 2,362 U.S. participants with hemochromatosis, the average amount of blood withdrawn during the initial phase of iron depletion was 33.9 units over an average time of 12.9 months. During maintenance therapy, the average amount of blood withdrawn was 1.7 units over an average time of 3.4 months.

Seventy-six percent said they had full or partial insurance coverage for therapeutic phlebotomy; 39 percent had no out-of-pocket payments. The average out-of-pocket payment per unit of blood was $45, but this figure includes those who claimed no charge at all. For those who paid for treatment, the average charge per unit of blood was $74 with a median charge of $50. The range went from $1 to $600. Average charges were as follows.

Hospitals:	*$90*
Physician's offices:	*$69*
Blood centers:	*$52*
Patient's home:	*$48.*

Phlebotomies are pretty cheap compared to other medical procedures—$75 to $100. And my insurance covers 80 percent of that.

I paid $30 to $35 for the first 60 units of blood I gave over a period of 40 years. Then the director of our local blood bank came to our support group meeting and told us that there was nothing wrong with our blood. He said that if we met all the other requirements for blood donation, he'd take us as donors.

It's great for me. I would still pay, but they don't let you. At my blood bank, it's free.

Under certain circumstances, people with hemochromatosis now may donate blood for transfusion and receive free phlebotomy. In August 1999, the Food and Drug Administration (FDA) issued a new ruling about blood donation. Blood banks may use blood from therapeutic phlebotomies of people with HH for transfusion (assuming the blood meets standard FDA criteria) if they don't charge for the phlebotomies and if they apply to the FDA for a special exemption, called a variance.

Before you visit your local blood bank, be sure to contact it to find out whether it has filed for the FDA variance (see Chapter 9 for more information).

RESOURCE: The American Hemochromatosis Society Web site lists blood banks with the FDA variance and other information. Web site: www.americanhs.org/bloodbanks.htm.

CHELATION COSTS. The iron-chelating agent approved in the United State is Desferal (deferoxamine mesylate). It is an expensive medication; treatment may cost thousands of dollars.

RESOURCE: Novartis Pharmaceuticals Corporation, the U.S. affiliate of Novartis AG, manufactures Desferal. Web site: www.pharma.us.novartis.com

RESOURCE: The Iron Overload Diseases Association Web site contains information on chelation costs. Web site: www.ironoverload.org/treatment.html

ONGOING MEDICAL CARE COSTS. If you have a chronic illness, like hemochromatosis, you have to consider the cost of lifelong medical care. When HH is diagnosed and treated early, you can prevent organ damage, but you will need regular exams, blood tests, and a regimen of phlebotomy treatments. On the other hand, severe hemochromatosis may require lifelong treatment for arthritis, heart disease, diabetes, liver disease, and hormonal problems.

What will it cost, for example, if you eventually need a solid organ transplant, such as a liver? According to Fabi Imo, Coordinator, Transplant Financial Services at the University of Colorado Health Sciences Center, the charges for liver transplantation (from admission to discharge, but not including before or after care) vary widely, from $50,000 to more than $1 million. The average charge is approximately $200,000. Costs vary widely around the country.

For help with transplant costs, work with your hospital transplant financial coordinator to explore all your options. Sometimes you have insurance benefits you're not aware of, such as coverage for travel, lodging, and mileage costs.

To get on the transplant list, I needed $120,000. Liver transplantation was still experimental in 1990 and not routinely covered by insurance. My situation was critical, so my wife and I began raising money.

People in my wife's company took up the cause, and then the company stepped in and covered my costs with their own insurance.

We probably could have raised the initial $120,000 on our own, but that didn't come close to covering the transplant. I was in the hospital for six months. It took half a million dollars.

BILL

According to Imo, sometimes patients who need financial help for liver transplantation find themselves in a Catch-22 situation. If you are disabled by liver disease and apply for Social Security Disability Insurance, a federal program, it takes 24 months (starting from the date you became eligible) for Medicare to become effective. Medicare does pay for liver transplants, but you may not be in a condition to wait two years.

"Another Catch-22 situation is the biggest problem I see," says Imo. "If the patient is over the minimum eligibility level, he or she will not qualify for Medicaid. And even if you have Medicaid, not all state Medicaid programs will cover a liver transplant."

Not all private insurance policies cover transplants. In addition, both private and government health insurance impose certain criteria. For example, people who have additional medical problems, such as a heart condition, a malignancy, or HIV, may find themselves excluded from coverage.

It's also important to look at your prescription drug benefit and how it covers immunosuppressive drugs. According to Imo, "The medications probably are the largest financial expense out of the patient's pocket. Post-transplant immunosuppressive medicines can be thousands of dollars a month." If you need help with medication costs, talk to your transplant coordinator about possible resources, such as pharmaceutical companies or state-funded social service programs.

My meds cost me—for two months worth—$30. The cost to my HMO is something like $900.

Right now my anti-rejection medicines cost about $235 a month. When I was first out of the hospital, they probably cost twice that. If I didn't have insurance, paying for my meds would be like an eternal car payment.

Medicare recently eliminated its former three-year time limit for coverage of post-transplant immunosuppressive medicines and now pays 80 percent of immunosuppressive drug costs for the lifetime of the transplanted organ. The patient must already be covered by Medicare at the time of transplantation. This policy applies to all Medicare entitled beneficiaries who meet all of the other program requirements for coverage under this benefit.

According to Imo, "A problem may occur when a patient is reassessed by the Social Security Administration and is no longer deemed disabled. Medicare is no longer effective, and the patient loses not only the Medicare coverage for insurance purposes but also, and most importantly, the immunosuppression coverage. It's a real dilemma."

Adding to direct costs are many indirect expenses. Patients sometimes forget to allow for organ recovery costs or travel and lodging for family members, childcare, and so on. Finally, cautions Imo, it's important for patients to be involved with insurance companies. Know the name and phone number of your case manager, and always inform your financial coordinator and your transplant team immediately if you change insurance companies.

RESOURCE: A booklet by the United Network for Organ Sharing (UNOS), *What Every Patient Needs to Know*, discusses a number of topics, including financing transplantation. For a copy, call 1-888-TXINFO1 (1-888-894-6361). You may also order on the UNOS Web site: www.unos.org.

RESOURCE: Another booklet, written by volunteers and distributed by the Organ Donor Program, may be helpful. For your free copy of *Finger in the Dike, Or: How to Raise $140,000 for Organ Transplant Surgery in Less Than Four Weeks,* call 1-800-452-1369 and ask for the Organ Donor Program.

RESOURCE: The American Liver Foundation (ALF) has established a Liver Transplant Fund that provides professional administration, at no cost, for funds raised on behalf of patients to help pay for medical care and associated transplantation expenses. For information, call 1-800-GO-LIVER or 1-888-367-4372.

Private Health Insurance

SELECTING PRIVATE HEALTH INSURANCE. When you have a chronic illness like hemochromatosis, you must select your health insurance carefully:

- *Read your policy before signing it. Ask questions. If there is any part you don't understand, get help.*
- *Make sure your plan allows you to see doctors who are experts in hemochromatosis: gastroenterologists, hepatologists, hematologists, and other specialists.*

- *Understand the restrictions and make sure they won't affect the quality of your care. For example, does the policy cover emergency rooms, experimental treatments, phlebotomies, drugs such as Desferal for chelation therapy? What happens if you're out of town and you need medical help?*

- *Is there a lifetime limit or cap on treatment or drugs? A million dollars may sound high, but is it too low for a chronic condition?*

- *Use common sense in assessing a medical policy. When you have hemochromatosis, you have to plan ahead for extra medical care, even though you may never need it.*

- *Check to see if your policy pays based on "reasonable and customary" fee schedules. Policies that use fee schedules may not pay the entire bill if they feel that your doctor or hospital does not charge "reasonable" rates.*

- *Know any managed care provisions in your policy. Do you have any particular doctor or hospital that you are required to use? If you use a "preferred provider," will the insurance cover a larger share?*

- *Become knowledgeable about the issues of genetic discrimination (see Genetic Discrimination and Insurance at the end of this chapter).*

TYPES OF PRIVATE HEALTH INSURANCE: MANAGED CARE OR FEE-FOR-SERVICE. Private health insurance policies fall into two categories: (1) managed care, or (2) fee for service. Managed care plans limit your choice of physician, but usually cost less. Managed care options include Health Maintenance Organizations (HMO) and Preferred Provider Organizations (PPO).

Fee-for-service policies usually provide the freedom to choose your doctor, but they often are more expensive. Consider the following factors when comparing cost of fee-for-service policies:

- MONTHLY PREMIUMS—*what the insurance costs each month.*

- ANNUAL DEDUCTIBLE—*how much you have to pay out of your pocket each year before the policy will pay benefits.*

- COINSURANCE—*what percentage you have to pay that your insurance will not cover, usually 20 to 30 percent.*

- OUT-OF-POCKET MAXIMUM—*the amount that you pay in coinsurance before the insurance company will begin to pay at one hundred percent.*

- POLICY MAXIMUM—*the maximum amount that insurance will pay over the lifetime of the policy.*

Whether you choose a managed care or a traditional fee-for-service plan, be sure you understand how your plan works and the appeal process. If you're dissatisfied with your insurance policy, you may always review these issues with your State Commissioner of Insurance.

HMOs. Under HMO plans you have a primary care physician, a gatekeeper, who coordinates your care and decides if you should be referred to a specialist. This plan is the least costly but the most limiting in terms of freedom of choice. Because the goal is to keep costs at a minimum, your access to specialists, tests, medications, or hospital care may be restricted. It's important to do a thorough check on limitations.

PPOs. You may choose a doctor within the provider network and get 90 to 100 percent coverage of your costs or choose a doctor outside the network and receive a smaller percentage of the cost, usually 70 percent.

Fee-for-Service Plans. Usually, the choice of doctor is totally yours, but these plans are typically the most expensive. Patients with hemochromatosis who are exploring fee-for-service plans should choose a major medical policy that offers subspecialty physician services and adequate hospital coverage.

The insurance company usually pays 80 percent of the bill, and you pay 20 percent up to a total amount designated by your policy. Hospital and physician fees that the insurance company deems unreasonable may not be fully reimbursed.

RESOURCE: To help consumers with the process of choosing a suitable health-care plan, check out two government Web sites: the Quality Interagency Coordination Task Force at www.consumer.gov/qualityhealth/index.html and the Department of Health and Human Services at www.healthfinder.gov.

RESOURCE: For help evaluating health insurance plans, call the National Committee for Quality Assurance at 1-800-839-6487 or 1-888-275-7585 for a personalized list of accredited HMOs in your area or visit its Web site to view *Choosing Quality: Finding the Health Plan That's Right for You* (archives section): www.ncqa.org

RESOURCE: Another useful booklet is *Checkup on Health Insurance Choices*, AHCPR #93-0018, by the Agency for Health Care Policy and Research: 1-800-358-9295.

RESOURCE: In 1996, Congress passed the *Health Insurance Portability and Accountability Act* (Public Law #104-191), sponsored by Senators Edward Kennedy and Nancy Kassebaum. This act includes many significant health insurance reforms. Some highlights of the act include: (1) "portability" provisions, (2) increased availability of coverage, and (3) expansion of the Consolidated Omnibus Budget Reconciliation Act of 1985 (COBRA) continuation coverage benefits. The "portability" provisions are designed to eliminate the fear that employees will lose their health insurance if they change jobs.

COBRA covered me for eighteen months when I was laid off at age 57 and decided to retire. I called the various big companies for health insurance. But when I put down hemochromatosis—man, did I get a letter back. "Sir, we have to turn you down because of your pre-existing conditions."

I'm lucky that in my state, we have a system where there is a company that has to give you health insurance if you are uninsurable. But I believe the law allows them to charge you a premium over the average rates. I've been covered since 1997, but this year the premium was $6,000 and it's going up $100 a month next year.

TOM

You may request a copy of the act and its accompanying conference committee report from your U.S. representative or senator. Also, as with other legislation of this type, government agencies, such as the Labor Department, the Internal Revenue Service, and the Department of Health and Human Services, issue regulations to implement the act's provisions. In addition, almost all states made changes in state legislation to comply with the act. For information, call your state legislators and your state insurance department.

RESOURCE: For questions about the Health Insurance Portability and Accountability Act (HIPAA), contact the Centers for Medicare and Medicaid Services (CMS), located at 7500 Security Blvd., Baltimore, MD 21244-1850. Toll-Free Phone: 877-267-2323, TTY Toll-Free: 866-226-1819 HIPAA Hotline: 1-866-282-0659

The HIPAA Web site contains information regarding consumers, employers, state regulators, COBRA, etc. Web site: www.cms.hhs.gov/hipaa/

RESOURCE: Some states have set up risk-sharing pools to enable people who are otherwise uninsurable to purchase health insurance. State insurance laws differ, so call your state insurance department for specific information. If you have difficulty locating your state insurance department, contact the National Association of Insurance Commissioners for the listing: 816-842-3600. Web site: www.naic.org

For information on various states' high-risk insurance pools, access the Web site of the National Association of State Comprehensive Health Insurance Plans (NASCHIP): www.naschip.org/states_pools.htm.

RESOURCE: Insure.com is a consumer insurance guide Web site that explains your COBRA rights and your rights to health insurance portability under HIPAA. Web site: www.insure.com/health/cobra.html and www.insure.com/health/hipaa.html.

Government Health Insurance

CAUTION: Laws and regulations change over time. Double-check your facts with the agency involved. Only the agency itself can give you up-to-date, accurate material.

There are some situations in which Medicare may eventually end, based on Social Security Disability Insurance (SSDI) eligibility. Also, the effects of work on benefits [SSDI and Supplemental Security Income (SSI)] and Medicare/Medicaid are complicated and different depending on what benefit you get. The best thing to do is to call the Social Security Administration before you or your spouse works to see what the specific effects will be on your cash benefits and/or medical coverage.

This chapter does not give legal advice and is not a substitute for the professional services of an attorney. Always consult a lawyer when legal issues are involved.

MEDICARE. At age 65, you may be eligible for medical insurance for hospital and other medical services. If you receive Social Security disability benefits for 24 consecutive months (see following section), you also may qualify for Medicare.

Medicare has two parts. Hospital insurance (Part A) covers inpatient hospital care. You already paid for this as part of your Social Security and Medicare taxes when you were working. Medical insurance (Part B) pays for doctors' services, post-transplant immunosuppressants, and some outpatient facility and doctor visits. Part B is optional, and you'll be billed monthly for your premium.

If you are not already getting Social Security benefits, sign up for Medicare at your local Social Security office three months before you become 65, and you'll receive your Medicare card. Ask about enrollment periods. If you are getting Social Security benefits, you will automatically be enrolled, and you will receive your card in the mail. You may also want to purchase a Medigap policy, or HMO, or other Medicare supplement (private insurance that fills in some of the "gaps" in Medicare's coverage).

RESOURCES: For more information, call 1-800-MEDICARE, or access the Web site (www.medicare.gov) to read or order publications, such as *Medicare & You* and *Guide to Health Insurance for People with Medicare: Choosing a Medigap Policy.*

If you have a low income and few resources, you may qualify for state aid to help pay for Medicare premiums and some other expenses; ask for Guide to Health Insurance. You may also call the Department of Social Services.

MEDICAID. Medicaid is a federal-state health program for people with low assets and incomes. At present, state social services departments administer the program. To apply, call your county social services department.

VETERANS ADMINISTRATION (VA). For questions about medical benefits and disability, veterans may call the Veterans Administration Regional Office. Dial 1-800-827-1000 and your call will be automatically directed to your regional office:

When You're Too Sick to Work: Applying for Disability

With advanced stage hemochromatosis when organ damage has occurred, you may be less capable of functioning at home or on the job. Our goal in this section is to provide you with resources for researching disability benefits and the process involved. For those who wish to consider applying for disability benefits, the process varies depending on your income, personal situation, and insurers or government programs.

CAUTION:

1. Laws and regulations change; unexpected circumstances arise. It's best to double-check your facts with the company, agency, or organization involved. Medical social workers can help direct you to the appropriate agencies or programs.

2. Keep a file with copies of all your medical records. Begin right now, if you haven't already done so. Always keep your EOBs (Explanation of Benefits) sent to you by your insurance company. The EOB is the document that explains what the medical provider and/or hospital is paid and contains a description of payment procedures.

3. Start a journal. Keep track of your symptoms and how they affect your daily tasks. This documentation will help you explain your symptoms to your doctor and will be important later if you ever have to file for disability.

4. This chapter does not give legal advice and is not a substitute for the professional services of an attorney. Consider consultation with a lawyer when legal issues or hearings are involved.

RESOURCE: Call the American Bar Association at 312-988-5000 for your state's lawyer referral service number or check your phone book. Attorneys specialize in different areas, such as disability or insurance, so explain your specific problem. If you can't afford a lawyer, contact your local Legal Aid Society or a law school that sponsors a student association offering free legal advice. Your local United Way may also direct you to possible sources of legal help.

SHORT-TERM DISABILITY LEAVE. Become familiar with your company's policies. Some companies offer paid short-term disability leave or allow you to use accumulated sick days. Companies usually require that a doctor accurately assess the nature of your symptoms and verify that you are disabled.

If you are an eligible employee and you or your family member (child, parent, spouse) becomes seriously ill, the Family and Medical

Leave Act allows you to take up to 12 weeks of unpaid leave each year. Workers returning from leave must be restored to their original jobs or equivalent jobs with the same pay, benefits, and working conditions.

RESOURCE: For more information and to find out if you are an eligible employee under the act, call the nearest office of the Wage and Hour Division, listed in most telephone directories under U.S. Government, Department of Labor, Employment Standards Administration.

RESOURCE: The 1990 Americans with Disabilities Act (ADA) prohibits job discrimination against "qualified individuals with disabilities." Employers covered under the act must make a "reasonable accommodation" for such persons depending on the particular facts in each case and on whether or not it imposes "due hardship" on the employer. "Reasonable accommodations" apply to the area of attendance and leave policies. To see whether the ADA covers you and your employer and to get more specific information on the provisions of the act, call the President's Committee on Employment of People with Disabilities Job Accommodation Network at 1-800-ADA-WORK or 1-800-526-7234.; email:jan@jan.icdi.wvu.edu; Web site: www.jan.wvu.edu.

(For more information on the ADA, see the Genetic Discrimination and Insurance section later in this chapter.)

Disability Insurance Resources

I was raising two daughters by myself, so my first liver transplant put a strain on everybody. Good thing I had insurance. I wouldn't be alive without it. It covered most of my second transplant, but I'm still in the process of paying some large bills.

My insurance only partially covered the costs of procuring an organ and left me with a $15,000 bill. It didn't cover my meds, but I qualified for some assistance from the state. I'm trying my best to stay off disability. I don't want to lose my house.

LARRY

If you're self-employed, you may have paid for your own individual disability insurance. If you work for a company, find out if you are eligible to enroll in your company's group disability coverage. Read the terms of coverage carefully.

Two Social Security Administration programs offer assistance if you have to file for disability: Social Security Disability Insurance (SSDI) and Supplemental Security Income (SSI).

CAUTION: Brief descriptions of the programs follow, but only the agency itself can give you up-to-date, accurate material. *Call the Social Security Administration and ask that you be sent information about disability programs: 1-800-772-1213.* You can speak to a service representative (in Spanish or English) between the hours of 7:00 a.m. and 7:00 p.m. on business days. Hearing-impaired callers using TTY equipment can call 1-800-325-0778 during the same hours. Web site: www.ssa.gov

SOCIAL SECURITY DISABILITY INSURANCE (SSDI). This insurance covers workers (and their children or surviving spouses). To qualify for this disability coverage on your own record, you must have worked long enough and recently enough to have made sufficient contributions to your Social Security account. You may also qualify on the record of a parent or as a disabled widow(er). Adults must have a physical and/or mental problem that prevents them from working for at least a year or that is expected to result in death. Benefits continue until a person is able to work and earn a certain amount of money again on a regular basis.

> *I filed for SSDI, and until the diagnosis of HH came back, I was just hanging out there. It took six months for approval, and then months before the first check came. But the check was for nine months worth from the day I filed. Of course, I was disabled before that, but they only went back nine months.*

> *I got a disability qualification—SSDI. As a result, I qualified for Medicare, and so my HMO took me. It was good for me, but I'm not sure it was good for them.*
>
> *On the other hand, my fees, co-pay, and deductible for my meds go up every year. But I can't complain, because without the HMO, it would be an extreme financial hardship*
>
> *I spent a lot of time at the blood bank. They had a draw fee, a lab fee; it all came to $90. But my insurance covered it.*

You may file a claim by phone, mail, or by visiting the nearest Social Security office. The claims process can take about 180 days while the agency obtains medical information and decides if the disability affects your ability to work. Call the Social Security Administration for the SSDI pamphlets that describe the program and list the medical and work information you will be asked to provide. The Social Security Administration recommends that you don't wait to file your claim, even if you don't have all the requested information right away. (There is a waiting period before benefits begin, so the sooner you apply, the better.) If you need help, a family member, caseworker, or other representative can contact the agency for you.

If the claim is approved, you'll receive a notice showing the amount of your benefit and when payments start. The amount of your benefit is based on your lifetime average earnings covered by Social Security, but workers' compensation benefits can affect your disability check. Your case will be reviewed periodically to see if you remain disabled. After two years from the date of onset of disability, you will be eligible for Medicare benefits, regardless of your age. If your claim is denied, a notice will explain why, and you will have opportunities to contest the decision.

RESOURCE: Call the Social Security Administration at 1-800-772-1213 (Web site: www.ssa.gov). Talk to a representative and ask for all available SSDI pamphlets.

SUPPLEMENTAL SECURITY INCOME (SSI). SSI is a Social Security Administration program that makes disability payments to adults and children with little or no income or resources. To get SSI, you must be 65 or older, blind, or disabled. (Disabled means you have a physical or mental problem that keeps you from substantial work and is expected to last at least a year or to result in death.)

The basic SSI payment is the same all over the country, but some states add money to your check. Any income you or your spouse has may affect the check amount. Call the Social Security Administration for information.

If you qualify for SSI, in most states you will be able to get other aid from your state or county, such as Medicaid (which helps pay doctor and hospital bills), food stamps, or other social services. Call your local social services department or public welfare office.

If you get Medicare and have low income and few resources, you may qualify for help with some Medicare premiums or co-pays under the Qualified Medicare Beneficiary (QMB) or Specified Low-Income Medicare Beneficiary (SLMB) programs. Only your state can decide if you qualify. Contact your county Social Services.

Whether your income meets SSI requirements depends on some very specific criteria defining what's included in income and what's included as assets. For more information, call the Social Security Administration.

Sometimes people can get both Social Security and SSI benefits. The rules that determine whether you're disabled are the same for Social Security and SSI (refer to the previous section, Social Security Disability Insurance.) You must be unable to do any substantial kind of work to be considered disabled under both programs.

If you think you are eligible for SSI, the Social Security Administration recommends that you file a claim right away, even if you don't have all the information at hand. The SSI pamphlets list the information you will need to supply.

> RESOURCE: Call the Social Security Administration at 1–800–772–1213
> (Web site: www.ssa.gov). Talk to a representative and ask for all available SSI
> pamphlets.

Genetic Discrimination in Insurance and Employment

The issue of genetic discrimination is tied to medical privacy. Who has access to your medical information? What can they do with it?

Genetic information can be used positively when, for example, genetic tests alert family members to HH. But that information can also be used negatively to deny insurance coverage, to increase insurance rates, and to discriminate in hiring for fear of raising the costs of health insurance.

When an employment or insurance physical involves blood and urine testing, your genetic material becomes available. Of course, there is no way to determine exactly how many people are denied coverage or employment due to genetic discrimination, because companies may give other reasons for their decisions.

In a survey of thousands of HH patients published in 1999, 20 percent with severe hemochromatosis (compared to 3 percent without severe HH) reported job loss. Seven percent said that they had lost their health insurance because they were refused coverage or because increased costs were prohibitive. In addition, 7 percent were refused life insurance.

ARE THERE SAFEGUARDS AGAINST GENETIC DISCRIMINATION?
"Over half the states now have some type of legislation," says Carol Walton, M.S., C.G.C., Director of the Graduate Program in Genetic Counseling at the University of Colorado Health Sciences Center. "The problem is that the legislation is quite variable from state to state in terms of the type of insurance protected and how the genetic diagnosis was made.

"Colorado, for example, says that only certain kinds of genetic testing are protected. If you have a genetic test based on the direct testing of DNA, RNA, or chromosomes, it's covered under the law. But it's not clear whether the law still protects you if you had a diagnosis based on the testing of the protein made by the mutated gene. And the law does not include diagnoses made solely by clinical symptoms. Most people are diagnosed by screening with a gene product test, such as a ferritin test, rather than genetic testing. Also, the Colorado law covers only health care insurance, group disability, or long-term care insurance. Even then, some types of policies, such as those provided by self-insured groups that are not subject to the jurisdiction of the state insurance commissioner, are not included. Life insurance and individual disability insurance are also not included.

"For the most part," adds Walton, "these laws have not been tested in the courts. The difficulty is that you may be protected in one state, but you may subsequently move to another state and not be protected there. That's why federal legislation is so important."

At the time of this writing, Congress has not yet passed the federal Genetic Nondiscrimination in Health Insurance and Employment Act, which prohibits genetic discrimination by health insurers and employers.

Federal employees are legally protected against genetic discrimination by Executive Order 13145, which President Clinton signed on February 9, 2000. The order prohibits the federal government and its agencies from using results of genetic tests in any employment decision.

> RESOURCE: To read summaries of state legislation on genetic discrimination and to track federal policy, access the National Human Genome Research Institute (NHGRI) Web site, Policy and Legislation. Web site: www.genome.gov
>
> RESOURCE: For information about your state insurance laws, contact your state insurance department. If you need help locating the department, contact the National Association of Insurance Commissioners for the listing. Phone: 816-842-3600. Web site: www.naic.org

The Health Insurance Portability and Accountability Act of 1996 (HIPAA) contains some provisions that protect workers' health insurance coverage in the areas of portability and pre-existing conditions, although they are not specific to genetics. Contact the Centers for Medicare & Medicaid Services (listed in Resource section below) for up-to-date information about your particular situation.

Some HIPAA provisions relevant to people with genetic conditions (although they are not specific to genetics) include the following:

+ *No insurer or employer can exclude an employee/family member of an employer group from health insurance based on health status.*

+ *Once an insurer sells a policy to any individual or group, it is required to renew coverage regardless of the health status of any member of the group.*

+ *Certain individuals who lose group coverage because of loss or change of employment will be guaranteed access to individual coverage without regard to health status.*

+ *Workers covered by group insurance policies generally cannot be excluded from coverage for more than 12 months for a pre-existing medical condition. Such limits can be placed only on conditions treated or diagnosed within the 6 months prior to their enrollment in a group health plan, and group insurers and group health plans must credit against the length of any pre-existing condition exclusion the length of previous coverage a person had that was not interrupted by a 63-day break in coverage.*

RESOURCE: For more information on the above and other specific HIPAA provisions, access the Centers for Medicare & Medicaid Services (CMS) HIPAA Online, an interactive tool that answers questions about your rights under the Health Insurance Portability and Accountability Act: Web site: www.cms.hhs.gov/hipaa1

According to HIPAA Online, "Genetic information cannot be used by group health plans to deny or cancel your coverage or to apply a pre-existing condition exclusion to your coverage. However, if genetic information contributes to the diagnosis of a medical condition, a preexisting condition exclusion might be applied to your coverage."[1] Similarly, HIPAA Online states, "If a genetic test provides only genetic information, the results of the test cannot be used by a group health plan to deny you coverage or to apply preexisting conditions to your coverage. If a genetic test contributes to the diagnosis of a medical condition, a preexisting condition exclusion might be applied to your coverage."[2]

RESOURCE: For information about the Health Insurance Portability and Accountability Act (HIPAA), contact the Centers for Medicare and Medicaid Services (CMS), located at 7500 Security Blvd., Baltimore, MD 21244-1850. Toll-Free Phone: 877-267-2323, TTY Toll-Free: 866-226-1819 HIPAA Hotline: 1-866-282-0659 Email: askhipaa@cms.hhs.gov Web site: www.cms.hhs.gov HIPAA Online: www.cms.hhs.gov/hipaa1

The Americans with Disabilities Act of 1990 (ADA) affords some protection against genetic discrimination on the job. Genetic job discrimination is difficult to prove. Usually it occurs when a company, especially a small business, is reluctant to hire or keep you because of concern over the impact on health insurance costs.

Can genetic test results lead to job discrimination? In a recent legal victory, the Equal Employment Opportunity Commission (EEOC) settled a preliminary injunction against the Burlington Northern Santa Fe Railway for $2.2 million. It was the EEOC's first court action challenging genetic testing of employees by a private company under the Americans with Disabilities Act. The EEOC argued that genetic testing is prohibited by the ADA, which forbids employers from conducting non-employment related medical inquiries. The company denied any wrongdoing.

In this case, the railway tested blood samples of employees without the employees' knowledge or consent. The settlement was with 36 railway workers who had filed on-the-job injury claims for carpal tunnel syndrome, caused mainly by the repetitive motions involved in laying railway tracks. Burlington Northern had tested for a genetic marker for carpal tunnel syndrome, presumably to use the evidence of genetic links to deny paying benefits.

RESOURCE: For questions about the Americans with Disabilities Act (ADA), contact the Job Accommodation Network (JAN), a service of the Office of Disability Employment Policy of the U.S. Department of Labor, P.O. Box 6080, WVU, Morgantown, WV 26506-6080. Phone: 1-800-ADA-WORK (Voice/TTY) or 1-800-526-7234 (Voice/TTY) Email: jan@jan.icdi.wvu.edu; Web site: www.jan.wvu.edu

RESOURCE: A news release, "EEOC Settles ADA Suit Against BNSF for Genetic Bias," can be found on the Web site of the U.S. Equal Employment Opportunity Commission. Web site: www.eeoc.gov/press/4-18-01.html

Another concern people have about genetic discrimination concerns the ability to interpret genetic information accurately. Genetic tests, for example, are predictive; they predict the chances of developing HH, but they do not guarantee that people will actually develop HH. Are insurance companies and employers aware that people with HH who are diagnosed and treated early have normal life expectancies? Do they realize that people who are carriers almost never develop HH?

According to the results of a CDC survey questionnaire published in 1999, about 7 percent of people with HH reported that they had lost their health insurance, either because they were refused coverage or because the increase in cost was prohibitive. About the same percentage reported that they were refused life insurance. Although the percentages were lower for people without severe HH, the figures raise issues about whether insurance companies fully understand that when hemochromatosis is diagnosed and treated early, patients enjoy normal life expectancy.

Paul Seligman, M.D., Professor of Medicine at the University of Colorado School of Medicine, Division of Hematology and Oncology, describes a typical scenario. "A patient with hemochromatosis who has no organ damage is treated with phlebotomy. But the person changes jobs and may have a problem with insurance due to his medical records stating pre-existing conditions. I write a letter to the insurance company assuring them that the condition is being treated and that the patient will have a normal life expectancy."

The wave of legislation that occurred in the 1990s in the U.S. was a response to the number of reported cases of insurance discrimination based on genetic information, including denial of coverage, raising of rates, and limiting the extent of coverage. A U.S. study, published in 2000, evaluated the impact of state laws restricting health insurers' use of genetic information. After conducting in-person interviews with insurers and a direct market test, the researchers found that a person with a genetic condition who had no actual symptoms faced little or no difficulty obtaining health insurance. The authors concluded that although insurers and agents are only vaguely aware of the new laws, nevertheless the laws have decreased the likelihood of insurers using genetic information in the future.

The same researchers, however, also found that the genetic anti-discrimination laws did not reduce people's *fear* of genetic discrimination in health insurance. Less certain was the extent to which this fear kept people from ordering genetic tests. Fear played virtually no role in pediatric or prenatal genetic situations but was significant for adult-onset conditions. The cost of testing was also a factor, especially when people did not want to apply for reimbursement but could not afford to pay on their own.

"I think genetic discrimination is where the real problems may arise," says Dr. Seligman," rather than focusing on a small percentage of people who have significant life-threatening problems. Geneticists are now suggesting new terminology called genetic polymorphism, which means mild mutations that do not cause disease in the carrier state and may actually be beneficial. We're all walking around with mutations, and some of them may be beneficial."

RESOURCE: If you feel that you have experienced employment, health, disability and/or life insurance discrimination due to HH, you may want to participate in a discrimination survey conducted by the Genetic Alliance. Web site: www.geneticalliance.org/aboutus/discrimination1.html

This iron time
Of doubt, disputes, distractions, fears.
MATHEW ARNOLD
Memorial Verses

REFERENCES

1. *HIPPA Online,* 29 Aug. 2002, Centers for Medicare & Medicaid Services, "Can my group health coverage be denied or cancelled based on genetic information?" 17 Dec. 2002 <www.cms.hhs.gov/hipaa/online/420141.asp>.

2. *HIPPA Online,* 29 Aug. 2002, Centers for Medicare & Medicaid Services, "If I take a genetic test, can the results be used to deny or limit my coverage?" 17 Dec. 2002 <www.cms.hhs.gov/hipaa/online/420142.asp>.

9

TREATMENT FOR HEMOCHROMATOSIS

Phlebotomy and Other Issues

When you've got HH, you donate blood and get cookies and juice. That's pretty good compared to some diseases where they can't do anything for you.

Look at it this way. Blood cells live for 120 days before they die. You're donating every 56 days or so. Therefore, your blood cells on average are younger—so you're partly getting younger.

ARTHUR

WHEN I TELL PATIENTS THAT THE TREAT-
ment for HH is phlebotomy, they usually react with surprise: "Bloodletting? I thought that went out with the Middle Ages." Most people don't realize that bloodletting was a common medical practice until the mid-nineteenth century. Today, doctors prescribe phlebotomy to treat hemochromatosis.

Phlebotomy, the therapeutic practice of opening a vein, is simple, effective, and relatively inexpensive. But it's only human to feel protective about our blood, which is traditionally viewed as the essence of life. Therefore, we'll also present some historical facts and myths about blood. Of course, you and your doctor will work together to decide on a treatment plan, but it helps to demystify the process by learning as much as you can.

- *Overview*
- *Phlebotomy Facts from Ancient to Modern Times*
- *Phlebotomy Treatment*
    WHAT IS PHLEBOTOMY?
    HOW DOES PHLEBOTOMY REDUCE IRON?
    WHO SHOULD BE TREATED?
    PHASE 1: IRON DEPLETION THERAPY
    PHASE 2: MAINTENANCE THERAPY
    BENEFITS OF TREATMENT
- *Iron Chelation Therapy*
- *The Patient's Experience*
    OVERCOMING TREATMENT PROBLEMS
- *Treatment Tips from Patients*
- *Blood Banks and the FDA*

Overview

As a patient with hemochromatosis, you may experience some fatigue and loss of energy. In addition, perhaps you are nervous about starting phlebotomy treatment or concerned about lifelong monitoring of iron overload. If you've already suffered organ damage, you also must deal with difficult chronic conditions. These symptoms and feelings may make you emotional or susceptible to periods of depression.

I encourage you to continue to remain physically active, pursue your occupation, socialize, and maintain proper nutrition. I also recommend regular exercise and a well-balanced diet supplemented with one iron-free multivitamin per day. (See Chapters 6 and 7 for more detailed suggestions on how to take care of yourself nutritionally and emotionally.)

Phlebotomy Facts from Ancient to Modern Times

Blood keeps us alive. Your bloodstream delivers oxygen and nutrients to organs, hauls away waste, and creates antibodies to fight germs. Hemoglobin, a protein that carries iron, is in red blood cells. The iron helps the blood absorb oxygen and this mixture of iron and oxygen is what makes blood red. Adults have about nine (females) to twelve (males) pints of blood in our bodies—about 10 percent of our body weight.

Blood is so important to us that many blood-related expressions have entered our language: hot- or cold-blooded, blue-blooded, young blood, new blood, bloodthirsty, bloodlust, bloodbath, bloodsucker, blood brother, in cold blood, to have someone's blood on your hands, to sweat blood, to taste blood, to make one's blood boil, and so on.

SOME HISTORICAL FACTS AND MYTHS ABOUT BLOODLETTING: No one knows exactly when phlebotomy began, but the ancient Egyptians used it as far back as 2500 B.C. Hippocrates, who lived in ancient Greece and is called the Father of Medicine, wrote detailed descriptions about the therapeutic use of bleeding, especially for inflammation. Bloodletting was based on theories of body "humors" (the body being composed of four humors: blood, phlegm, black bile, and yellow bile). Health and disease depended upon the balance and imbalance of these four humors—hence the need to balance the body by drawing off excess blood.

Astrology often helped to determine the time of procedure, as the following lines from the *Regimen Sanitatis Salernitanum* indicate:

> *"Three special months, September, April, May*
> *There are in which 'tis good to ope a vein.*
> *In these three months the moon bears greatest sway."* [1]

The poem probably dates from the 13th century. A popular medical health code, it appeared in many languages and almost 300 different editions until 1846.

In the 14th century, the Black Death swept the civilized world, killing about a fourth of the population. In London, half the people died. Plague tracts written for the people suggested drinking vinegar—and bloodletting.

In America, in the 18th century, a controversial physican, Benjamin Rush, was a strong advocate of bloodletting. A brilliant man who graduated from Princeton at age 15, Rush was one of the signers of the Declaration of Independence. During the yellow fever epidemic in Philadelphia at the turn of the century, he insisted that yellow fever was not contagious and prescribed purges, enemas, baths, and bleeding. He started with 10 to 12 ounces of blood and increased the amount to 80 ounces in some cases. Protests against bloodletting, however, were increasing, and it was noted that Rush lost three of his apprentices and his own sister to these harsh methods.[2]

Finally, in 19th century France, a physician named P. C. A. Louis delivered the death blow to bloodletting as a regular form of therapy. He did it by what he called his Numerical Method—counting. Although the method seems obvious today, it was a revolutionary concept at the time. Louis observed 78 cases of pneumonia, 33 cases of erysipelas, and 23 cases of inflammation of the throat. Then he compared those bled to those not bled. When he found no difference in mortality, length of illness, or type of symptom, bleeding fell into disfavor.[3] During the last third of the 19th century, scientific advances and the discovery of bacteria contributed to the decline of bloodletting.

Today, people with hemochromatosis owe a great debt to Professor C. A. Finch of Seattle, who introduced therapeutic phlebotomy for the removal of excess iron in 1947.[4]

Phlebotomy Treatment

WHAT IS PHLEBOTOMY? Phlebotomy (derived from the Greek word for vein, phléps) is the practice of opening a vein for the therapeutic letting of blood. A phlebotomist is a nurse or health care worker specially trained to draw venous blood. Another word for phlebotomy is venesection (from the Latin venae sectio, the cutting of a vein). In contrast to the advances in molecular understanding of iron overload and the discovery of key mutations in the HFE gene, phlebotomy treatment is "low tech." It is also simple, inexpensive, and safe.

HOW DOES PHLEBOTOMY REDUCE IRON? Patients with hemochromatosis have increased blood ferritin, increased transferrin saturation, and often have high normal or elevated hematocrit (a measure of red cells). These three findings demonstrate the link between iron and blood cell production by the bone marrow. Excess iron supplied to the bone marrow maintains a higher level of red cells in the blood.

The removal of one unit of blood (500 milliliters) depletes the body of approximately 200 to 250 milligrams of iron. The removal of four to five units is required to deplete the body of 1 gram of iron.

Removing blood causes the release of hormones, primarily erythropoeitin, that stimulate the bone marrow to produce more blood (erythropoeisis). During the process of forming new blood the body must supply additional iron.

Patients with hemochromatosis have extremely high total body iron, which is stored primarily as tissue ferritin and hemosiderin. Blood ferritin level is a crude marker for tissue iron stores: the higher the blood ferritin, the larger the tissue pool of stored iron. As the formation of new blood accelerates to replace the blood lost through phlebotomy, iron is pulled from the tissues where it has been stored.

A large number of phlebotomies are typically required to deplete body iron in adult patients with hemochromatosis. Take the case of a man age 50, just recently diagnosed with HH. On average, he could be expected to have approximately 20 grams of total body iron. It will take 80 to 100 phlebotomies to deplete his body of iron! That's one phlebotomy per week, with intermittent rest periods, for nearly two years.

WHO SHOULD BE TREATED? The evidence for use of phlebotomy in the treatment of hemochromatosis is overwhelming. When instituted prior to the onset of cirrhosis or diabetes, phlebotomy virtually eliminates these complications, prevents other organ damage due to iron overload, and restores a normal state of health. Early identification of asymptomatic cases of HH and phlebotomy for those with evidence of iron overload is required. However, even symptomatic patients, or those with organ damage can benefit from iron depletion.

Iron overload sufficient to institute treatment is defined by transferrin saturation greater than 45 percent with elevated ferritin. Phlebotomy, without performance of liver biopsy, is indicated in patients younger than 40 years, ferritin less than 1000 ng/ml, and normal liver enzymes. Older patients, or patients with ferritin over 1000 ng/ml or abnormal liver enzymes, need liver biopsies to stage fibrosis and detect cirrhosis. (See Chapter 2 for descriptions of transferrin, ferritin, biopsies, etc.)

A liver biopsy (for tissue iron concentration) may be useful in patients with compound heterozygosity (C282Y/H63D). In these patients the blood tests for iron overload may be elevated, but tissue iron levels may be normal. Results from the biopsy could guide decisions regarding phlebotomy treatment.

In general, phlebotomy is not indicated in patients with transferrin saturation less than 45 percent who also have normal ferritin.

PHASE 1: IRON DEPLETION THERAPY. The goal of depletion therapy is to reduce the body's stores of iron to the normal range. Because a single phlebotomy removes only 0.2 to 0.25 grams, two to three years of weekly phlebotomy are required to deplete 20 to 30 grams of iron from the body. Some have advocated twice weekly phlebotomy to accelerate the process of iron removal. However, this regimen can be inconvenient, tedious and difficult for many patients.

Complications of cardiac involvement, including arrhythmias and heart failure, may worsen during rapid mobilization of iron. Vitamin C may accelerate the mobilization of iron from tissue stores and increase risks in patients with cardiac disease. For these reasons, slower rates of iron depletion (no more than one phlebotomy per week) and the avoidance of supplemental vitamin C is recommended for the patient with cardiac hemochromatosis.

When iron is depleted, the production of red blood cells by the bone marrow decreases. Hematocrit is determined prior to each phlebotomy, and phlebotomy is performed as long as the hematocrit has not fallen by more than 20 percent from its prior level. For example, if the initial hematocrit is 50, you would proceed with the next phlebotomy as long as the hematocrit is greater than 40. For patients with lower starting hematocrits, other lower limits of hematocrit for the performance of phlebotomy may be applied, such as an absolute hematocrit of 38 percent.

The simplest indicator of body iron depletion is the failure of the hematocrit to recover prior to the next phlebotomy. However, measurement of ferritin approximately every 10 to 12 phlebotomies provides additional information. Once the ferritin level has dropped to 50 ng/ml it is likely that all excess iron stores have been mobilized. Dropping ferritin levels below 25 ng/ml should be avoided as this indicates iron deficiency. Obviously in the latter circumstance, phlebotomy must be put on hold.

PHASE 2: MAINTENANCE THERAPY. Even though you can be depleted of iron within two to three years by frequent phlebotomy, iron stores will ultimately re-accumulate if phlebotomy ceases. The goal of maintenance phlebotomy is to maintain normal iron stores and prevent re-accumulation of excess iron. The frequency of maintenance phlebotomy varies among patients, depending upon the individual's rate of iron re-accumulation. Some may require monthly phlebotomy, whereas others may require phlebotomy only every four months. Many factors may contribute to the varying rates of re-accumulation of iron after iron depletion: dietary iron intake (iron containing supplements, excessive intake of red meat), use of alcohol, supplements containing vitamin C, age, gender, and other biological or genetic variables related to the molecular events of iron absorption by the intestine. The goals of maintenance therapy are to keep the hematocrit in the low normal range and maintain ferritin between 25 to 50 ng/ml.

BENEFITS OF TREATMENT. Clearly a major goal is to identify cases of HH prior to organ damage and clinical complications. Institution of iron depletion and maintenance treatment in these individuals restores a normal state of health and prolongs life.

However, symptomatic patients, including those with organ damage from iron overload, also benefit from iron depletion. Some clinical features consistently improve, including a sense of well-being and a lessening of fatigue and skin pigmentation. Often insulin requirements in diabetics will diminish, and abdominal pain or discomforts will lessen.

Other features of HH, such as arthritis, cirrhosis, and impotence, are less responsive and may not significantly improve. Liver cancer remains a threat in patients with underlying cirrhosis, even after iron depletion.

Patients with end-stage hemochromatosis may require liver transplantation. Infectious and cardiac complications after liver transplantation in HH patients may be related to excessive iron stores at the time of transplantation. Some have advocated iron depletion prior to transplant to reduce these complications, but the effectiveness of this strategy is unproven.

Iron Chelation Therapy

This treatment is used mainly in secondary forms of iron overload, related to the use of transfusions to treat anemia. In this clinical setting, transfusions are given to maintain the hematocrit, and removal of blood by phlebotomy is not indicated and is potentially dangerous. Large numbers of transfusions lead to marked accumulation of iron in the body, which can result in organ damage and clinical complications similar to those that occur in hemochromatosis.

Because phlebotomy is not an option, medications were developed that bind iron (chelators), removing it from tissues and delivering it to the kidney for excretion into the urine. The most commonly used iron chelator is deferoxamine.

Although it has been used in clinical practice for nearly 20 years, deferoxamine has several drawbacks. It must be administered intravenously, usually as a continuous infusion over twelve hours, four to six days per week. Treatments are time-consuming and uncomfortable, and many patients are poorly tolerant of the side effects. Side effects can include local skin reactions, hearing loss, nerve damage, lung damage, and local infections at infusion sites.

One other agent, deferipone, has been developed as an oral agent. Initial studies suggested that this agent was similar to deferoxamine in its ability to mobilize and remove body iron. However, a long-term study of deferipone in patients with secondary iron overload indicated that it was ineffective in preventing iron overload and hepatic damage. Additional studies will be required to determine the role of deferipone as an iron chelator.

Iron chelation therapy is not usually recommended for patients with hemochromatosis.

The Patient's Experience

The blood donation process takes about 20 minutes. You lie down or sit in a reclining chair. The phlebotomist cleanses the skin on the inner part of the elbow joint, and a new, sterile needle is inserted into an arm vein. The needle is already connected to plastic tubing and a blood bag. You may be asked to squeeze your hand to help blood flow from the vein into the blood bag. Usually, one unit of blood, about one pint, is collected.

Your body replaces the fluid lost from donation in 24 hours. It takes up to two months to replace the lost red blood cells.

A survey of phlebotomy therapy among HH patients, published in 1999, reported some interesting results from 2,362 U.S. participants. More than 77 percent reported that they believed the treatment was beneficial; 15 percent voiced a negative opinion about therapy; 59 percent said that if they could take a pill with a 5 percent risk of side effects, they would prefer the pill to phlebotomy. Patients mentioned the following main negative points: difficulty accessing a vein, time involved (travel, waiting, the procedure), and the fact that the blood was not used for donation.

OVERCOMING TREATMENT PROBLEMS. As noted above, weekly phlebotomy can be a "drag." Patients complain that the process of phlebotomy is inconvenient, cumbersome, tedious, and occasionally difficult, especially when access to a vein (venous access) is a problem.

Several simple suggestions may improve the phlebotomy experience. Take in extra fluid beginning the day prior to and day of phlebotomy. If you are sick, dehydrated, or suffering from gastrointestinal upset with nausea, vomiting, or diarrhea, cancel and reschedule your phlebotomy appointment. Discuss your concerns with the phlebotomist, and review your treatment with your physician. It helps to remind yourself, or have others remind you, that the treatment is effective at eliminating or reducing the long-term clinical problems associated with untreated hemochromatosis.

Treatment Tips from Patients

My dad and I walked into the clinic and rolled up our sleeves. That was the beginning of treatment for both of us. He went one time a week; I went one time a month.

I didn't do so well, but I got smart. As the blood was leaving my body, I'd drink juice.

I'm petite, five feet tall on a good day. I had a lot of anxiety about phlebotomies, and that added to my difficulties. I had a reaction. I'd get nauseous and pass out. It was a nightmare for two days after.

I learned to ask for a smaller gauge needle—a 21 gauge, rather than a 16 gauge.

When I was de-ironed in May 2000, I got my period regularly for the first time in my life—and I've been regular ever since. Now I get a phlebotomy every 56 days.

I had so many headaches that I never made it three weeks without one. They knew me in the emergency room. I didn't even have to check in. As my iron came down with phlebotomies, I had fewer headaches.

I worry about my veins wearing out by the time I'm 50.

A friend of mine with HH said that after a phlebotomy, he felt like he got hit by a bus.

I try to drink a half-gallon of water before a phlebotomy, and it makes a great deal of difference. I drink water afterwards, too. I always eat salty food right before. It helps because it makes me thirsty—so I drink more.

One time I drank tea all day. When I got to the blood bank, they said, "You've been drinking a lot of caffeine today." Tea dehydrates you. It took a little longer to get the blood out.

I had pseudo-arthritis, deposits of iron compound in my joints—not calcium. After weekly phlebotomies for 38 weeks, I got back to normal and my "arthritis" disappeared. My liver and spleen returned to normal size, too.

The beautiful thing about my blood donation is it's free. And they treat you like a king. When you have to go anywhere else for medical procedures, it's scary.

After my coma and diagnosis for HH, I spent some 60 weeks getting phlebotomies to get the iron down. I say it didn't affect me, but it did. I tried to stay positive.

The nurses were terrific. They kept my spirits up. Instead of making it an ordeal, they were positive and upbeat. I wouldn't want to do it again, though.

After a while, my veins started to scar up, and my arms were a mess. The nurses just kept working to find veins. There was no choice. They were as glad as I was when my levels went down.

I'd have two phlebotomies the week before my vacation. And I wouldn't be out of town more than a week—so I kept my average of one a week.

I became a blood-making factory. I had blood taken every three days for 44 weeks. No one without HH could have endured such a rigorous phlebotomy schedule without having iron overload, because they would have become seriously anemic.

It was really weird. Bloodletting is medieval—like going back to using leaches. But maybe medieval treatments had some science behind them, because some viruses, like hepatitis viruses, love iron.

After my forty-second phlebotomy, I started to think that I couldn't do it anymore. I'd have to stop midway on a flight of stairs. I just couldn't cope. But the next time I went, the doctor said, "You're done." Now I have maintenance treatments every two to three months. My body told me when to stop.

Once I started weekly phlebotomies, my headaches stopped. I'd had them since childhood, and they were debilitating the last few years. Imagine a sinus headache magnified, a three- to four-hour deal. They'd start behind my eyes or on one side of my head and gradually grow. I'd have to make arrangements when a headache would start, because I couldn't do anything. I couldn't work.

My hair started coming back with the phlebotomies, I no longer notice my slight heart arrhythmia, but my joint pain is the same.

I was like a zombie. I used to be articulate, but I couldn't remember words. After phlebotomies de-ironed me, I was tremendously better.

Needles have always scared the hell out of me because of my army experience. I was 22 years old and had just gotten my shot. I was at the end of the line. We all fell in and marched off. Suddenly I saw stars and blacked out. I fainted on the parade ground. Then I got up and ran after my outfit.

Since then, needles just really affect me. Thirty years later, I had to get a phlebotomy every week. I was sweating, trembling. My face was pure white. But I got so I became very comfortable with it. I almost looked forward to it because I got friendly with the phlebotomists.

Who likes to get stuck with needles? But everyone benefits. You get rid of the blood, and at my blood bank people that need the blood get it. You have to have a positive outlook about it.

Blood Banks and the FDA

About 60 percent of Americans are eligible to donate blood, but only 5 percent do so.[5] Blood shortages, therefore, are a continuing national problem. HH blood is iron-rich and healthy, so why not add it to the nation's blood supply?

Until recently, the FDA did not prohibit the use of blood from therapeutic phlebotomies, but the blood had to be labeled with the donor's disease. Needless to say, this practice discouraged the use of HH blood for transfusion.

> *It's the word disease. If you call HH a disease, the blood banks don't want people to think they're using diseased blood. It's a public relations thing. Any doctor or expert would say it's okay to use HH blood.*

> *I've been getting a phlebotomy at a blood bank every two months. I had to pay them to throw my blood away. It took a long time for them to learn that nothing is wrong with HH blood.*

"You were always allowed to collect the blood, but you had to identify it with a label of hereditary hemochromatosis. There was no reason not to use it, but recipients were reluctant to use blood that came from people with some kind of disorder," says Hannis W. Thompson, M.D., Director of Transfusion Medicine at the University of Colorado Medical School and Associate Professor of Pathology.

In August 1999, the Food and Drug Administration (FDA) issued a new ruling concerning blood collection and donation. Blood banks may use blood from therapeutic phlebotomies of people with HH for transfusion (assuming the blood meets the standard FDA criteria, of course) if they don't charge for the phlebotomies and if they apply to the FDA for a special exemption, called a variance, from existing regulations.

The variance provides guidelines for blood banks (1) that wish to distribute blood collected from people with HH without indicating the disorder on the label, and (2) that wish to collect blood from people with HH more frequently than every 8 weeks. (Call your blood bank for specific information about prescriptions or check the Web site resources below.) The blood banks must offer free phlebotomy to HH patients. In addition, the blood banks must collect and submit safety data to the FDA.

Under the variance, no hemochromatosis donor will be charged for a phlebotomy even if the donor does not qualify to be a routine blood donor after a history and physical examination. This eliminates a possible incentive for a donor to deny risk conditions that might prevent a cost-free donation.

Note: Before you visit your local blood banks, be sure to contact it to find out whether it has filed for the FDA variance.

RESOURCE: The American Hemochromatosis Society Web site features an updated list of blood banks that have received a variance from the FDA. In addition, the site has information about the FDA rule, a sample letter that patients can send to their blood bank for free treatment, a sample letter that the blood bank has to submit to the FDA to receive a variance, and the FDA approval letter. Web site: www.americanhs.org/bloodbanks.htm

RESOURCE: To obtain a copy of the FDA's "Guidance for Industry, Variances for Blood Collection from Individuals with Hereditary Hemochromatosis," contact the Office of Communication, Training and Manufacturers Assistance, (HFM-40), Center for Biologics Evaluation and Research (CBER), Food and Drug Administration, 1401 Rockville Pike, Rockville, MD 20852-1448. Phone: 1-800-835-4709 or 301-827-1800; Web site: www.fda.gov/cber/gdlns/hemchrom.htm

For the life of the flesh is in the blood ...
LEVITICUS *17:11*

REFERENCE

1. Douglas Guthrie, *A History of Medicine* (Philadelphia: J. B. Lippincott Co., 1946) 109.
2. Louis Lasagna, M.D., *The Doctors' Dilemmas* (New York: Harper & Brothers, 1962) 51-57.
3. Lasagna, 14.
4. Wintrobe, Maxwell M., M.D., Ph.D., M.A.C.P., hon.D.Sc. *Blood, Pure and Eloquent* (New York: McGraw-Hill, 1980) 177.
5. "National Blood Supplies Critically Sparse," *The Denver Post.* June 28, 2002: 6A.

10

LIVER CANCER (HEPATOMA)

Are You at Risk?

I started to retain fluid in my legs and stomach. My urine was brown. My eyes were yellow.

I had been a heavy drinker. After tests and a biopsy, the doctor found three things: hemochromatosis, that I once had hepatitis B, and cirrhosis of the liver. Along with the drinking, all three things cooked my goose. That day I took my last drink.

"I have good news and bad news," my doctor said. "The bad news is you have liver cancer. The good news is we caught it early."

EVAN

MOST OF MY PATIENTS DON'T REALIZE THAT hemochromatosis can cause liver cancer (hepatoma). But before you panic or worry unnecessarily, consider the following:

1. Only a minority of patients with hemochromatosis will ever develop liver cancer.
2. Effective therapies exist for tumors detected early.
3. Liver cancer is almost entirely restricted to those with advanced liver disease who have extensive fibrosis (stage III or IV) or cirrhosis.

Of course, you're wondering if you are in danger. This chapter provides you with information regarding risk factors, warning signs, screening and diagnostic tests, and results of current treatment. Here are the topics I'll cover:

- *Overview: What Is Liver Cancer?*
  PRIMARY LIVER CANCER (HEPATOMA)
  SECONDARY LIVER CANCER
  RISE IN LIVER CANCER IN THE U.S.

- *Common Risk Factors*
  STAGE OF LIVER DISEASE
  AGE, DURATION OF IRON OVERLOAD, IMPACT OF
    IRON UNLOADING
  OTHER LIVER DISEASES

- *Warning Signs*
  NO SYMPTOMS BUT WITH UNDERLYING CIRRHOSIS
  DETERIORATION IN LIVER FUNCTION
  PAIN
  SUDDEN DEVELOPMENT OF PORTAL HYPERTENSION
  OTHER SYMPTOMS

- *Testing*
  EARLY SCREENING GUIDELINES
    (1) Blood Tests (Serial Measurement of Alpha-fetoprotein)
    (2) Radiologic Imaging
  DIAGNOSTIC TESTS

- *Treatment*
  CANCER STAGING
    (1) Early Stage
    (2) Advanced Stage
    (3) Metastic Liver Cancer
  HEPATIC RESECTION
  TRANSPLANTATION
  CHEMOEMBOLIZATION
  HIGH-FREQUENCY RADIO WAVES (RADIOFREQUENCY
  TUMOR ABLATION)
  ALCOHOL INJECTION, CRYOSURGERY
  CHEMOTHERAPY

- *A Word About Cancers Beyond the Liver*
- *Summary*

Overview: What Is Liver Cancer?

PRIMARY LIVER CANCER (HEPATOMA). Primary liver cancer, also known as hepatoma or hepatocellular carcinoma, is a malignant tumor that originates within the liver. In the United States, primary liver cancer is relatively rare, compared to cancers of lung, breast and colon.

SECONDARY LIVER CANCER. When I interview patients they often tell me that a relative died of "liver cancer." On further questioning, I learn that the person actually first had a cancer in another location within the body, such as the colon, but then died later after the cancer had spread to the liver. Cancers that have spread from another site to the liver are termed secondary liver cancers. Secondary liver cancers are more commonly encountered in clinical practice than primary liver cancers and often appear as multiple masses, while primary liver cancers typically appear as a solitary mass.

> *When I was a kid, my mom was in the hospital all the time for all kinds of stuff. She had colon cancer and then developed liver cancer. It was inoperable.*
>
> *My doctor thought she died from hemochromatosis. People weren't testing and looking for HH then.*
>
> JAN

Physicians distinguish secondary from primary liver cancers by imaging (ultrasonography, CT, MRI) and biopsy of the liver. The finding of secondary liver cancer means that tumor cells have traveled far from their primary site, typically indicating a poor chance of survival. Liver transplantation is not indicated for secondary liver cancers.

RISE IN LIVER CANCER IN THE U.S. Twenty to 30 years ago, primary liver cancer was rare in the United States. I remember attending medical case conferences as a student or resident when the focus of the presentation was the rare, unique, or atypical occurrence of hepatoma. Although hepatoma was rare in the U.S. at that time, it was a common cancer and a leading cause of cancer-related death in Asia and Africa due to a high prevalence of viral hepatitis.

Today, we diagnose primary liver cancer with increasing frequency in this country. The Centers for Disease Control and Prevention reported that the incidence of hepatoma increased from 1.4 to 2.4 per 100,000 people between 1979 and 1995. In my own state of Colorado, the number of cases of hepatoma doubled from 1988 to 1998. The number of patients with hepatoma presented to the Tumor Board at University Hospital was 6 in 1988 and 24 in 1997.

The increase in liver cancer in the U.S. is related primarily to chronic hepatitis C. There is no evidence that the rise in incidence of hepatoma is linked independently to hemochromatosis. However, patients with hemochromatosis who also have hepatitis C may be at particularly high risk for hepatoma.

> *I've got HH and hepatitis C. One night I wound up reading a book about hepatitis C at 1AM, but I didn't read the chapter on liver cancer. That's not going to happen, I thought.*
>
> *Well, I ended up reading the chapter, and it said hemochromatosis with hepatitis C can lead to liver cancer. I said, "Oh my God. I never thought of that.*
>
> *I had put my head in the sand. I got really scared—so I finally went on treatment for hepatitis C.*
>
> LANI

Common Risk Factors

STAGE OF LIVER DISEASE. The most important predictor of liver cancer is the condition of the liver tissue (histologic stage). Patients who lack significant fibrosis have a low risk, patients with extensive fibrosis run an intermediate risk, and those with cirrhosis are at greatest risk.

A recent study from Italy examined the risk of hepatoma in 230 patients with hemochromatosis followed for an average of 80 months. At baseline, 134 had cirrhosis and 96 were non–cirrhotic. Forty-nine patients developed hepatoma, and all were in the cirrhotic group. None of the patients without cirrhosis developed hepatoma. The average age of the patients who developed hepatoma was 59 years. This information suggests that the annual risk for developing hepatoma in a patient with hemochromatosis and cirrhosis is approximately 5 percent per year [(49 hepatomas/134 cirrhotics) x (100%) x (1/(80 months/12 months in a year))].

Other reports indicate that from 20 percent to as many as 45 percent of deaths in patients with hemochromatosis and cirrhosis are due to hepatoma, a risk that is 100- to 200-fold higher than the general population. Hepatoma may develop in cirrhotic patients even after iron depletion.

There are 13 reported cases of hepatoma occurring in noncirrhotic patients, but most of these patients had substantial fibrosis. Existing reports indicate that HH patients without significant fibrosis are at low risk for hepatoma and screening for liver tumors is not recommended. In contrast, patients with cirrhosis run a considerable lifetime risk of developing hepatoma and should undergo screening with serial determination of alpha-fetoprotein and liver imaging. Cirrhotic patients who develop sudden onset of decompensation (see Chapter 5) should undergo diagnostic studies to rule out liver cancer.

AGE, DURATION OF IRON OVERLOAD, IMPACT OF IRON UNLOADING. The sequence of events that transforms normal liver cells into cancer is not completely defined. Multiple steps may be required, including iron accumulation, liver injury, formation of fibrosis, and evolution to cirrhosis. The average age of patients with hemochromatosis who develop cancer ranges between 55 to 65 years, approximately 10 years older than the average age for development of cirrhosis.

Three findings indicate that development of cirrhosis is a key step in the development of hepatoma. First, nearly all cases of hepatoma in hemochromatosis occur in patients with cirrhosis. Second, hepatoma risk is still very high in cirrhotics, even after iron depletion. Third, patients without significant fibrosis or cirrhosis who undergo iron depletion therapy do not develop cirrhosis or hepatoma. Risk of cirrhosis is due, in turn, to the duration and severity of iron overload.

Iron itself may promote the formation of cancer. The risk of liver cancer in hemochromatosis patients was compared to the risk of cancer in patients whose liver disease was caused mainly by alcohol or viral hepatitis. The two groups had similar stages of liver disease. Interestingly, HH patients were nearly twice as likely to develop hepatoma as the non-HH group (relative risk 1.8). Because the two groups were well matched in terms of extent of fibrosis or percent with cirrhosis, the increased risk in HH patients was thought to be due mainly to iron overload.

Effects of iron overload that potentially contribute to cancer formation include the promotion of oxidant injury and the impairment of immune functions. The fact that risk of cancer persists even after iron depletion, suggests that the effect of iron on the development of cancer may occur at earlier steps in cancer formation.

OTHER LIVER DISEASES. Because cirrhosis is clearly linked to the risk for hepatoma in patients with hemochromatosis, any liver disease that hastens the development of cirrhosis may also increase the likelihood of developing hepatoma. The three most common concurrent hepatic diseases in hemochromatosis are alcoholic liver disease, viral hepatitis, and non-alcoholic fatty liver.

Study results indicate that patients with HH who drink alcohol add fuel to the hepatoma fire. Chronic daily consumption of alcohol is associated with acceleration to cirrhosis, increased risk for liver failure, increased risk for needing liver transplantation, and increased risk for development of liver cancer. Others have reported similar effects in patients with hemochromatosis who are infected with either hepatitis B or C.

> *I got disabled from the railroad because of arthritis. Two years later, I caught meningitis, and I started feeling fatigued. I was sleeping 15 to 20 hours a day, but I didn't want to believe I was sick.*
>
> *The Friday before Christmas, my doctor told me I had cancer in my liver. The biopsy showed too much iron in my body. I'm heterozygous for HH.*
>
> *I knew something wasn't right with me. I got my transplant six months later. I haven't rejected, but I have high levels of hepatitis C.*
>
> JUAN

In general, heterozygotes who carry one mutation of either C282Y or H63D are not at risk for hepatoma. However, early results suggest that heterozygotes infected with either hepatitis C or hepatitis B may develop modest iron overload and increase their risk for hepatoma. Additional studies of risk of hepatoma in heterozygotes are needed.

TABLE 10. FACTORS ASSOCIATED WITH RISK OF LIVER CANCER (HEPATOMA)

CIRRHOSIS
IRON OVERLOAD (NOTE: RISK IN CIRRHOTICS IS NOT ELIMINATED BY IRON DEPLETION)
AGE > 50 YEARS
CHRONIC ALCOHOLISM
TOBACCO SMOKING
VIRAL HEPATITIS (B AND C)

Warning Signs

NO SYMPTOMS BUT WITH UNDERLYING CIRRHOSIS. Many patients develop hepatoma without any changes in symptoms or obvious progression of their disease. That's why screening tests, such as alpha-fetoprotein and ultrasonography, are often recommended for all patients with bridging fibrosis (stage III) or cirrhosis. Detection of hepatoma with screening tests may result in more effective treatment and better outcomes.

> *My mom was 63 when she went to the doctor because her hip hurt. That was her first symptom of hemochromatosis. She was limping because her hip joint had just rusted out.*
>
> *By the time she was diagnosed, she already had cirrhosis from HH—and that let to liver cancer. During her lifetime, she had 106 phlebotomies.*
>
> DELLA

DETERIORATION IN LIVER FUNCTION. A stable cirrhotic patient may be fully employed, have normal levels of energy, conduct normal social activities, and have stable liver tests. When such a patient develops hepatoma, liver function may deteriorate for no other apparent reason. Signs of deterioration are increasing fatigue, mental confusion (encephalopathy), fluid retention (ascites, edema), or gastrointestinal bleeding. Alternatively, the patient's liver tests may suddenly deteriorate with rising bilirubin, diminishing clotting factors, increase in liver enzymes, and drop in serum albumin. Some patients experience only a loss of appetite, fever, and unexplained weight loss.

PAIN. A tumor can grow rapidly, causing the liver capsule to expand, and tumor cells can invade adjacent nerve roots, blood vessels, and lymphatics. As the hepatoma enlarges and impinges on adjacent structures, it can create significant pain and discomfort. The development of persistent moderate to severe pain in the right upper quadrant of the abdomen in a patient with cirrhosis may point to the diagnosis of hepatoma.

> *Ten years before my husband was diagnosed with hemochromatosis, he had high liver enzymes. The doctor never did anything. My husband had kidney stones, gout, stomach trouble, broken bones…*

In 1991, it really got serious. He fell to the floor for no reason. We got him to the doctor, and a liver biopsy proved he had HH. It took two years to get his ferritin down from 2100 to 137.

I feel he should have been diagnosed earlier. He wouldn't be at the point he is now with the right side of his liver all cirrhosed.

Six weeks ago he wasn't feeling well. His readings were high. He lost 10 pounds, and had a horrendous pain in his abdomen. He said he felt his stomach was just stuck. A CT scan and ultrasound showed a big mass on the right side of his liver. A tumor the size of a quarter was pressing on his bile duct. They inserted a stent, and that helped for a while, but six weeks later, he was in the hospital again with an infection.

"No way I'm going to let them do anymore for a few, extra days with a poor quality of life," he said. So now we have home hospice care to control the pain with morphine. He's not eating well…

KRISTY

SUDDEN DEVELOPMENT OF PORTAL HYPERTENSION. Hepatoma is a vascular tumor and often invades vascular structures, such as blood or fluid-bearing vessels or ducts. If the tumor enters the portal vein, it may plug the vessel or cause blood clotting that blocks the vein. An acute rise in portal pressure related to this blockage may result in an upper gastrointestinal bleed (variceal hemorrhage), swelling of the abdomen (ascites) or ankles, worsening of existing ascites, development of diuretic-resistant ascites, mental confusion (encephalopathy), or worsening of existing encephalopathy.

OTHER SYMPTOMS. Patients may attribute certain nonspecific symptoms (fatigue, loss of appetite, poor energy) to their hemochromatosis when the symptoms may be related to emergence of hepatoma. These patients often delay notifying their physicians for several months. Such a delay may convert a potentially treatable tumor to one that has spread beyond the confines of the liver and may no longer be treatable.

Testing

EARLY SCREENING GUIDELINES. Doctors have not yet established guidelines for screening for hepatoma in patients with hemochromatosis. However, recent clinical trials have indicated that screening with both alpha-fetoprotein and ultrasonography detects early tumors and results in improved patient survival. Nonetheless, many of my comments on screening come from my own experience and represent my bias regarding the most cost-effective and sensitive approach to this problem.

Again, I want to emphasize that most patients with hemochromatosis will not develop primary liver cancer. Noncirrhotic patients appear to be at an exceedingly low risk, and only those with advanced fibrosis or cirrhosis who have had the disease for more than 20 years are at excess risk. Therefore, all comments regarding screening apply only to patients with bridging fibrosis (stage III) or cirrhosis.

The two types of screening tests doctors use to detect liver cancer are: (1) blood tests (serial measurement of alpha-fetoprotein) and (2) radiologic imaging.

(1) Blood Tests (Serial Measurement of Alpha-fetoprotein). Hepatoma cells synthesize a protein called alpha-fetoprotein and release the protein into the bloodstream. A very high alpha-fetoprotein [>500 nanograms (ng) per milliliter (ml)] or a sustained rise in alpha-fetoprotein on serial measurements (with the last value > 150 ng/ml) may predict the development of hepatoma. A subtype of alpha-fetoprotein (L3) may be more specific for cancer. Other blood tests, such as PIVKA-II, are under investigation.

The accuracy of alpha-fetoprotein, used alone, in predicting hepatoma is poor. Therefore, doctors may order supplemental radiologic tests, biopsies, or even a surgical incision (laparotomy). In addition, approximately one-third of the hepatomas that occur in patients with hemochromatosis don't produce alpha-fetoprotein, and the tumors progress undetected by the serial alpha-fetoprotein measurements. Radiologic imaging of the liver is required to screen for these tumors.

(2) Radiologic Imaging. Although CT scans and Magnetic Resonance Imaging (MRI) with enhancing agents may be slightly more sensitive than ultrasonography, they are prohibitively expensive for use in screening. Ultrasonography, on the other hand, which can detect the majority of early hepatomas, is much less costly and is the radiologic screening choice. I currently advise my cirrhotic patients and those with extensive fibrosis to have alpha-fetoprotein measurements every 6 months and ultrasonography of the liver at least annually.

DIAGNOSTIC TESTS. If screening tests detect a lesion that might be cancerous, doctors may biopsy the mass with the guidance of ultrasonography or CT (see Figure 10). Other imaging studies (CT, MRI, or angiography) can detect early hepatoma in the patient with rising alpha-fetoprotein or worsening of symptoms when ultrasonography fails to reveal a definite lesion. The type of imaging study is ordered at your physician's discretion.

FIGURE 10:

CT (COMPUTED TOMOGRAPHY) SCANS FROM AN UNAFFECTED INDIVIDUAL (LEFT) AND A PATIENT WITH HEMOCHROMATOSIS AND LIVER CANCER (RIGHT)

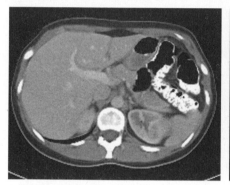 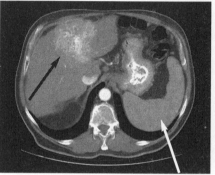

UNAFFECTED INDIVIDUAL   HEMOCHROMATOSIS WITH LIVER CANCER

LEGEND 10: *The liver of the unaffected individual is shown on the left. The liver from the patient with hemochromatosis was cirrhotic on liver biopsy. The mass (black arrow) is a biopsy-proven liver cancer. The spleen (white arrow) is enlarged as a result of cirrhosis.*

Treatment

CANCER STAGING. In order to select proper treatment, the physician must determine the stage of the hepatoma. This is usually done with radiologic imaging, laparoscopy, or abdominal exploratory surgery.

(1) Early Stage. Patients with a solitary tumor less than 5 centimeters in diameter or patients with up to three tumors, all less than 3 centimeters in diameter, may be candidates for surgery to remove the tumor (hepatic resection) or liver transplantation. Recurrence of the tumor is common if resection is performed. Cure and excellent long-term survival are the rule with liver transplantation.

(2) **Advanced Stage.** More advanced stages of hepatoma usually represent multiple tumor nodules involving one or both liver lobes. The tumor may have invaded the main liver vessels. Advanced stage tumors have a poorer prognosis, and typically doctors do not advise resection or transplantation. Most patients cannot undergo resection due to the extensive nature of the disease and the risk of precipitating liver failure because of underlying cirrhosis. Only a small subgroup is considered for transplantation. However, the outcome after liver transplantation is poor for patients with advanced stage hepatomas, because of recurrence of cancer. Patients with advanced stage cancer are considered for palliative treatment with either chemoembolization, cryosurgery, or radiofrequency thermal ablation.

(3) **Metastatic Liver Cancer.** Patients with widespread tumors that have metastasized (spread) beyond the confines of the liver are not candidates for surgery, transplantation, cryotherapy, or chemoembolization. They are evaluated only for standard chemotherapy.

HEPATIC RESECTION. Surgeons achieve the best results in the treatment of hepatoma when they perform a liver resection to surgically remove a solitary tumor (less than 5 centimeters) in a patient with a noncirrhotic liver. These patients may be cured of their cancer and usually enjoy long-term survival.

However, this represents an uncommon clinical scenario when it comes to hepatoma in patients with hemochromatosis. As I have already mentioned, the patient with hemochromatosis who develops a liver cancer usually has cirrhosis and is older, between the ages of 55 to 65.

Unfortunately, cirrhosis precludes a successful resection because resections for hepatoma usually require removing 25 to 75 percent of the liver tissue. A normal liver can tolerate a massive resection since regeneration is rapid (usually within 12 weeks) and the remaining liver cells are functioning normally. That's not the case when a person has cirrhosis. The remaining liver cannot effectively regenerate, and its function is severely impaired. When a surgeon performs a large resection on a cirrhotic patient, the operation may lead to liver failure. For these reasons liver resections are usually restricted to patients without cirrhosis or to those cirrhotic patients who have no evidence of clinical or biochemical deterioration in liver function or portal hypertension.

TRANSPLANTATION. Results from a number of centers agree. Cirrhotic patients with solitary liver cancers, small in size (less than 5 centimeters in diameter) or up to three tumors (all less than 3 centimeters in diameter), should be considered for transplantation.

> *I get a CT scan every two years to check on my transplant for liver cancer. I just had one, and everything is perfect. I pretty well take it in stride. My family is somewhat that way, too.*

> *Yeah, it was kind of sobering. I focused on the word "cancer." The hemochromatosis was kind of a sideline.*

> *The hemochromatosis was overshadowed by liver cancer. My doctor told me I had a couple of years left.*
> *They did a thorough job of pre-testing me for a transplant—three months of testing in order to make sure that the cancer was isolated. If it spreads to other organs, they won't transplant you. Four years ago, I had my transplant.*

Successful transplantation may also be performed on patients with multiple tumor nodules (all less than 2 centimeters) that are restricted to one hepatic lobe with no evidence of invasion of blood vessels. Although these two groups of patients can expect long-term, tumor-free survival, those with advanced stages of hepatoma or metastatic disease almost uniformly experience early post-transplant recurrence of tumor and death from metastatic disease. Transplantation is not indicated for the latter patients.

Even for hepatomas in favorable stages, time can run out. Most of the data that deals with successful transplants for hepatoma come from an era of relatively greater availability of donor livers. That situation no longer exists in this country. The U.S. waiting list for liver transplantation continues to expand. In December 2002, more than 17,000 people were on the list, but only about 4,500 liver transplants were performed that year.

Patients with hepatoma are at a distinct disadvantage as they wait for a liver. The tumor will grow with time, spread to adjacent areas of the liver, invade blood vessels, and prevent the patient from continuing as a transplant candidate. Patients with hepatoma are currently given higher MELD scores but may also need to be considered for living-donor liver transplantation (see Chapter 11).

Given current statistics, many have projected that by the year 2015 the U.S. waiting list will have over 30,000 patients. A sizeable number will develop hepatoma while waiting for a donor liver.

CHEMOEMBOLIZATION. This procedure does not cure cancer. However, it can help destroy local tumors, reduce the tumor mass, provide significant relief, or in the case of a solitary tumor, keep the tumor from spreading outside the liver until a donor liver becomes available.

> *I had a chemical treatment. They went with a tube through the artery near the groin and through the liver to cut off the blood supply that was supplying the cancer. That's one of the ways they were able to determine that it was the only cancer I had. And they treated it to stop the growth.*
>
> JAY

The technique involves placing a catheter through a vessel in the groin (the femoral artery) and advancing it into the liver's main artery (the hepatic artery). Then a special form of chemotherapy is infused through the catheter into the artery feeding the tumor. Both normal and hepatoma cells take up the chemotherapy, but cancer cells do not excrete it. Because cancer cells retain the chemotherapy for a prolonged time, they are destroyed.

Although chemoembolization may be used as a bridge to resection or transplantation, chemoembolization alone is rarely, if ever, curative. In the absence of resection or transplantation, spread or recurrence of the cancer is the rule. Despite these shortcomings, chemoembolization has been associated with prolonged survival and reduced symptoms of pain and weight loss. In transplant candidates, chemoembolization may sustain the patient until successful transplantation can take place.

HIGH-FREQUENCY RADIO WAVES (RADIOFREQUENCY TUMOR ABLATION). This treatment of hepatoma remains under study. The technique involves CT-guided puncture of the hepatoma and positioning the prongs of a special instrument within the tumor mass. High-frequency radio waves (near the microwave limit) generated within the tumor mass destroy the tumor. The overall effectiveness and clinical outcome of this treatment for hepatoma remain to be defined.

ALCOHOL INJECTION, CRYOSURGERY. These two approaches are also limited to hepatomas that cannot be resected or transplanted. The goal of these treatments is to reduce tumor size and relieve painful symptoms.

Alcohol injection is done with the guidance of a CT scan to ensure proper placement of the treatment catheter within the tumor. Absolute alcohol (ethyl alcohol containing less than 1 percent water) dehydrates the tissues, causing the immediate death of cells, and starts a clotting process within the tumor that destroys it.

Cryosurgery involves the use of a flexible fiberoptic instrument (laparoscopy) with the guidance of an ultrasound probe to properly position the cryosurgical instrument within the tumor. When the probe is positioned, the tumor cells are destroyed by freezing.

CHEMOTHERAPY. Hepatoma is one of the most resistant tumors to both radiation and chemotherapy. Early experience with external beam radiation suggested that doses of radiation required for effective anti-tumor activity exceeded safety standards. In addition, clinical experience with radiation therapy of hepatomas has been mainly disappointing. Newer techniques using specialized forms of radiation, precise focusing of the beam within the tumor, and use of radiosensitizers are under investigation. One technique employing ferromagnetic beads impregnated with chemotherapy and external magnetic field focusing is currently in clinical trials. Some evidence suggests that systemic chemotherapy can be partially effective in reducing tumor burden and relieving symptoms.

A Word About Cancers Beyond the Liver

At the time of this writing, there were a limited number of studies regarding the risk of nonhepatic malignancy in patients with hemochromatosis. One study compared the risk of nonhepatic malignancy in 230 HH patients to a matched cohort of patients with other liver diseases. Twenty HH patients and 11 non-HH patients developed nonhepatic malignancies during 80 months of follow-up. This difference did not reach statistical significance, but there was a trend toward greater risk in the HH patients (relative risk 1.8, statistically not significant). The nonhepatic malignancies included tumors of the colon, pancreas, lung, prostate, and breast.

Patients with HH do not develop unique or unusual tumors and there are no unique or HH-specific screening guidelines. The current recommendation is simply to follow standard screening guidelines for the general population regarding detection of the common malignancies.

Summary

Primary liver cancer is an extremely serious, life-threatening complication of hemochromatosis, but it occurs mainly in patients with advanced disease and cirrhosis. Patients with bridging fibrosis or cirrhosis should be aware of the danger of liver cancer, undergo screening by their physician, and know the warning signs.

Early hepatoma is treatable, but most patients with large tumors or multiple tumors cannot be treated by liver resection or transplantation. Cirrhotic patients with solitary and small hepatomas should be considered for early liver transplantation and possibly living-donor transplantation. A number of new approaches can reduce but not cure inoperable tumors: chemoembolization, radiofrequency thermal ablation, alcohol ablation, cryosurgery, and systemic chemotherapy.

Liver cancer is an increasingly important issue for HH patients, families, physicians, surgeons, transplant programs, and the health care system in general. We in the medical community know that we sorely need new ideas and new treatments.

It is always good
When a man has two irons in the fire.
  FRANCIS BEAUMONT AND JOHN FLETCHER
  The Faithful Friends

11

LIVER TRANSPLANTS FOR HEMOCHROMATOSIS

A Medical Miracle

I went from being perfectly healthy to almost dead in one year. I was hanging on by my nails. Everything started to go haywire. A biopsy showed my liver was in cirrhosis because of hemochromatosis. In six months I went from skiing and working to being deathly sick.

They started bleeding me extensively. They took blood every week for weeks on end. But it was way too late. So I was put on the transplant list.

HAROLD

SOME PEOPLE WITH HEMOCHROMATOSIS DEVelop cirrhosis, liver failure, and need a liver transplant to survive. Liver transplantation is the most complicated therapy for people with end-stage hemochromatosis, but it can produce seemingly miraculous results.

Pre-transplant patients go through a difficult time. They suffer from a variety of symptoms, including jaundice, sleeplessness, itching, fluid buildup, mental confusion, and hemorrhaging. A successful transplant cures these symptoms, and the patient can lead a full, productive life.

This chapter covers the following topics:

- *Liver Transplantation: A Brief History*
- *Who Gets a Liver Transplant?*
  TRANSPLANTS FOR PATIENTS WITH HEMOCHROMATOSIS
  SIGNS THAT YOU NEED A TRANSPLANT
  DENIAL OF TRANSPLANTS
  PAYING FOR TRANSPLANTS
- *The Transplant Team*
- *Waiting for a Liver*
  THE EVALUATION PROCESS
  THE WAITING LIST
  TRANSPLANT SUPPORT GROUPS
- *Liver Transplant Surgery*
  DONOR LIVERS
  LIVING-DONOR LIVER TRANSPLANT
  THE SURGICAL PROCEDURE
  THE HOSPITAL STAY
- *Living with a New Liver*
  MEDICATIONS TO PREVENT REJECTION
  MANAGING COMPLICATIONS
  PSYCHOLOGICAL TRANSFORMATION
- *Improved Survival Rates*
  OVERALL OUTCOME AFTER LIVER TRANSPLANTATION
  OUTCOME IN PATIENTS WITH HEMOCHROMATOSIS
- *Issues in Liver Transplantation for the Carrier (C282Y Heterozygote)*
- *How Organs Are Allocated*
  UNOS
  LISTING STATUS
  CENTERS OF EXCELLENCE

Liver Transplantation: A Brief History

The first liver transplant was performed by Dr. Thomas Starzl in 1963 at the University of Colorado in Denver. Twenty years later, in 1983, a National Institute of Health (NIH) consensus conference on the therapeutic role of liver transplantation concluded, "After extensive review and consideration . . . liver transplantation is a therapeutic modality for end-stage liver disease that deserves broader application."

At that time, only 6 centers in North America and 4 in Europe performed hepatic transplantation. Ten years later, 3,442 patients had the procedure at 88 centers in the United States. In December 2002, there were more than 17,000 patients on the active U.S. waiting list.

Who Gets a Liver Transplant?

TRANSPLANTS FOR PATIENTS WITH HEMOCHROMATOSIS. Liver transplantation is the most successful therapy for patients with a wide array of diseases that ultimately result in liver failure. Hemochromatosis is the most common inherited disorder in adults for which liver transplantation is performed. Alcohol or infection with either hepatitis B or C accelerates injury and speeds the progression of liver disease. Occasionally, heterozygotes who also have alcohol-induced liver disease or viral hepatitis may develop advanced disease and require liver transplantation.

SIGNS THAT YOU NEED A TRANSPLANT. Obvious clinical signs and symptoms usually accompany advanced liver disease, including:

- ASCITES *(accumulation of fluid in the abdomen);*
- ENCEPHALOPATHY *(alteration of mental function);*
- VARICEAL HEMORRHAGE *(bleeding from veins in the esophagus or stomach);*
- WORSENING NUTRITIONAL STATUS;
- DIMINISHING QUALITY OF LIFE.

Patients who have a spontaneous infection in the ascites fluid, low serum albumin (< 2.8 grams/deciliter), clotting problems (prothrombin time > 5 seconds prolonged), and severe sustained jaundice should be given urgent consideration for transplantation. All of the above findings indicate severe liver dysfunction and are late signs of end-stage liver disease.

Many people with cirrhosis have few or no findings of liver disease. Doctors say that these patients have "compensated" cirrhosis, and that it may be too early to consider liver transplantation. However, the waiting list for liver transplants is expanding, while the pool of donors is staying about the same. Patients often wait on the list for 1, 2, or more years before they get a liver.

Once you have cirrhosis, your doctor must monitor your blood tests closely and watch for any physical signs of decompensation in order to time the referral for liver transplantation. Unfortunately, not all patients with compensated cirrhosis are the same; some will remain stable for several years, but others may deteriorate relatively rapidly.

> *I got sick when I was 45 years old. I started coughing up dark blood that looked like coffee grounds. At the hospital, the doctor said I was an alcoholic and that I would die unless I quit drinking. I quit alcohol the next day. No big deal, but it wasn't the problem*
>
> *I quit for two years—and I coughed up coffee grounds again. My doctor said, "Are you drinking?" And I said, "Not a drop!" He didn't believe me, and he called me a "noncompliant patient."*
>
> *It was touch and go in intensive care. I had 3 to 4 bandings in three days. Then I was banded once a week for six to seven weeks.*
>
> *My liver enzymes were high. My red blood cell count was real high. Finally, a doctor said, "I know what's wrong with you—hemochromatosis. I had no idea what he was talking about. I had never heard of it.*
>
> ROGER

The course of hemochromatosis varies greatly, so your physician must make an imperfect estimate of your chances of having a life-threatening complication over a one- to two-year follow-up period. If your doctor estimates that you have more than a 10 percent chance of sustaining a complication within one year, you should be evaluated for transplantation.

DENIAL OF TRANSPLANTS. Liver transplants are typically denied in cases of active HIV infection or AIDS, incurable cancer, active infection in the blood, active alcohol abuse, or severe underlying heart, lung, or multi-organ disease. If you are elderly, morbidly obese, or have had prior extensive abdominal surgery, a clotted portal vein, extensive liver cancer, an isolated liver cancer larger than 5 centimeters, or cancer of the bile ducts, you might also be excluded from transplantation.

PAYING FOR TRANSPLANTS.   (See Chapter 8, Taking Care of Yourself Financially.)

The Transplant Team

Liver transplantation is a complex procedure requiring many specialists to care for you. Usually, your transplant team consists of a hepatologist, a hepatology nurse, a transplant surgeon, a transplant anesthesiologist, a transplant nurse coordinator (who keeps you informed and tells you when a liver becomes available), a social worker (who provides you and your family with emotional support), a psychiatrist (who meets with you and your family to evaluate your strengths and weaknesses and make recommendations to help you through the transplant experience), a nutritionist (who deals with pre-transplant issues, such as overweight problems or nutritional wasting, and helps with recommendations for your post-transplant nutritional needs), and a financial coordinator. Your outcome may be improved if your liver transplant program has a "team" approach and performs more than 20 transplants a year.

Waiting for a Liver

THE EVALUATION PROCESS. You will be asked to take many diagnostic tests and meet with a psychiatrist and social worker. Usually, you meet with each person on the transplant team. The process can take a couple of days. When all the tests and interviews are completed, the team meets to approve or deny your candidacy for transplantation and may suggest additional evaluations or consultations.

In trying to evaluate your ability to tolerate transplant surgery, the transplant team will give you some diagnostic tests. Depending on your condition, the tests may include blood tests, colonoscopy (view of the entire colon through a colonoscope), CT scan (a radiologic test that lets doctors see the anatomy and size of your liver), ECG (an electrocardiogram), endoscopy (a procedure that allows doctors to look for ulcers, masses, varices, or bleeding in the esophagus or stomach), ERCP (a procedure performed when there is concern about blockage or narrowing in the bile ducts), flexible sigmoidoscopy (a procedure that lets the physician look at the lower colon for polyps, hemorrhoids, ulcers, and colon or rectal cancer), pulmonary function tests (a breathing test that measures the function of your lungs), and ultrasound (a test that gives information about the size and shape of your liver through sound waves). If you have conditions that require additional tests, you may be asked to meet with a consultant, such as a cardiologist.

I had a three-day evaluation to get on the liver transplant list. It was amazing—and sort of fun. I never got so much attention in my whole life. It felt like I donated my body to science, even though I was still alive.

Some of it was weird. They didn't put me on a treadmill to test my heart. Instead, they gave me drugs to speed up my heartbeat and put me on monitors. The advantage is that they can actually observe things in me passively, instead of my having to move. It wasn't pleasant, but it was not uncomfortable. It was strange to be artificially stressed like that.

They gave me a psychological evaluation, a socioeconomic evaluation along with the complete physical. Because of the situation of limited resources, they want people who can handle the stress of post-transplant living, and who can stick to the regimen.

MEL

THE WAITING LIST. As previously noted, the number of patients on the waiting list continues to expand. Current patients placed on the list can wait for more than 2 years for a donor liver. This is an incredibly difficult and apprehensive period. While waiting, you may have to deal with life changes, physical symptoms, and financial changes. If you're the major breadwinner who can't go to work, you may lose the social network from your job.

A diminishing number of patients are transplanted in stable condition. Increasingly, transplants are performed in sicker patients who are hospitalized or in intensive care (see MELD score under How Organs Are Allocated, Listing Status).

It's critical at this stage to talk with a good friend or therapist about your struggles. Keeping a personal journal is helpful. You are going through a fundamental shift in how you think of yourself and preparing for the psychological changes of the transplant.

My doctor said I'm stable. I've been on the transplant list for seven years. Right now I'm too stable for the new guidelines. But I may get too old for a transplant.

I try to stay positive and not worry about something I can't do anything about anyway. I try to stay close to a 13 ferritin level. If it goes above that, I do a pull—a phlebotomy. They "pull" the iron out.

I've been waiting for a liver for seven years. My energy level is pretty good. I'm up at 6:30 and ready to go, but I don't have the stamina I had at 50. Now I limit my physical work to five or six hours a day.

If things become more critical, I might think about a living donor— but not now.

I was in the hospital after a car accident, when they discovered I had hemochromatosis. They were going to remove my gallbladder and started doing all these tests. Then they said they couldn't take it out because I'd bleed to death. I needed a liver.

I was on the waiting list for a year During that time I had a gastrointestinal bleed and was in a coma for nine days. I got pneumonia and was on intravenous therapy for six weeks. I had to have hearing and blood tests every three days because of an antibiotic. Both my inner ears were destroyed. It screwed up my balance.

The transplant waiting list is a list you don't want to be on. But if you have to be on it, you want to be on the bottom of the list. That means you're less damaged. I'm hoping for the miracle of regenerating tissue.

I try to keep a positive attitude while I'm waiting for a liver. I do what the doctor tells me to do, and I keep positive about it. You can beat yourself to death the other way.

TRANSPLANT SUPPORT GROUPS. Transplant support groups can be a source of strength and encouragement for pre- and post-transplant patients. The long waiting period, difficult symptoms, the trauma of surgery, the psychological shift of accepting another person's organ—all of these issues are unique to transplant patients. No one else can truly understand what it's like.

Your transplant team can refer you to a support group, or you can check the resources listed at the end of this chapter. In addition to support groups, many people tell me they find it helpful to read about other liver transplant patients' experiences and about the procedure itself. Here are some books my patients recommend:

RESOURCES:

Green, Reg. *The Nicholas Effect, A Boy's Gift to the World*. Sepastopol, Calif.: O'Reilly, 1999.

Maier, Frank with Ginny Maier. *Sweet Reprieve.* New York: Crown, 1991.

McCartney, Scott. *Defying the Gods.* New York: Macmillan, 1994.

Schomaker, Mary Zimmeth. *Life Line, How One Night Changed Five Lives.* Far Hills,. N.J.: New Horizon, 1996.

Starzl, Thomas E. *The Puzzle People.* Pittsburgh: University of Pittsburgh, 1992.

Liver Transplant Surgery

DONOR LIVERS. Liver transplantation is made possible only through the act of organ donation. In most states, you can sign an organ donor permission statement on your driver's license; a witnessed signature is a legal form of consent. Most organ procurement organizations, however, request additional consent from the closest living relative. These organizations identify potential donors by interacting with emergency rooms and intensive care units.

Organ donation is one of the highest forms of giving and caring, and the vast majority of religious denominations endorse it. The generosity of organ donation makes possible the miracle of transplantation.

Did you know that the liver donor usually donates as many as seven organs for seven different patients? Suitable liver donors are patients under age 65 who are brain-dead but whose hearts are beating. (In some cases, donors as old as 80 have been used.) They have no underlying malignancy, and they test negative for AIDS and active hepatitis B. The donors must have stable heart function with acceptable liver tests, serum sodium less than 170, and preferably been hospitalized for fewer than seven days. Donors and recipients must have compatible blood types and approximately similar body size but do not have to be of the same sex.

It's customary to biopsy the donor liver to be certain that it is not scarred, fatty, or severely damaged. Once recovered, the donated organs are flushed with a special solution that preserves them for up to 48 hours.

Despite efforts to use all potential donor organs, we currently face a crisis in supply and availability of donor organs. We encourage all readers of this book to work with their local organ procurement organizations to increase public awareness of the critical need and value of organ donation. It's important for all family members to discuss organ and tissue donation. Everyone should consider signing a Uniform Donor Card.

RESOURCE: For more information on organ donation, contact the Coalition on Donation, an alliance of national organizations and local coalitions that educates the public about organ donation, 700 N. 4th St., Richmond,VA 23219. Phone: 804-330-8620; Email: coalition@shareyourlife.org; Web site: www.shareyourlife.org

How can we as physicians attempt to deal with the crisis in availability of donor organs? The cadaveric supply of donor livers has remained relatively constant at about 4000 to 4500 donor livers each year for the last five years. The current U.S. waiting list is over 17,000.

We need to increase the donor pool in innovative ways in order to meet the expanding need for donor organs. Use of older donors and livers with increased amounts of fat has failed to substantially expand the donor pool. Splitting of cadaveric livers for use in two recipients works well for a pediatric (left lateral segment) and adult recipient (right lobe + left medial segment); splits for two adult recipients works less well. For this reason, our center and many others have embarked upon the use of adult living donors (right lobe donation) for adults.

LIVING-DONOR LIVER TRANSPLANT. You may be thinking, "By the time I need a transplant, there will be too many people on the waiting list, and I won't ever get one." One solution for the shortage of donors may be living-donor liver transplantation, where a portion of the donor's liver is removed and then transplanted. The Japanese, for example, still debate the concept of brain death so most liver donations in Japan are from live donors. In the past, the majority of live donor transplant operations were performed in pediatric recipients. Currently in the U.S., however, more live donor liver transplants are performed in adult than pediatric recipients.

At the time of this writing, the University of Colorado had performed more than 80 adult-to-adult live-donor liver transplantions with the vast majority between relatives, although close friends and personal relationships may be considered. All donors are alive and tolerated the liver resection. Their livers regenerated back to normal size within 16 weeks.

We recently evaluated the impact of right lobe donation on the quality of life of the living donors:

- *75% of donors recovered completely and returned to normal life within an average of 3.4 months after surgery.*
- *96% returned to work at an average of 2.4 months.*
- *42% described a change in body image related to the scar from the incision.*

+ *71% had mild ongoing abdominal discomfort.*

Personal relationships between donor and recipient were the same or better in 96 percent of cases. The relationship of the donor to his or her life partner was the same or better in 80 percent of cases. Most donors reported out-of-pocket expenses not covered by insurance plans. All patients reported that under the same circumstances they would donate again, and 96 percent of the donors felt that they benefited from the experience.

Survival and rates of retransplantation in recipients of living-donor liver transplants are similar to results after cadaveric transplants. Biliary complications occur more frequently compared to standard cadaveric transplantation. However, because of the critical lack of cadaveric donor livers, it is my opinion that living-donor donation for adults will become increasingly common in the United States.

In our program, we have developed selection criteria for both donor and recipient. Our current criteria for selection of recipients center around two concepts. First, we feel that recipients should have an excellent chance for favorable post-transplant outcome. Second, the recipient should be in urgent need of a transplant for survival and might die while waiting for standard cadaveric transplantation.

Donors for living donor liver transplantation must be relatively young (younger than 50 years old), normal body size, healthy without medical problems, and they cannot have a history of prior abdominal surgery. Donors and recipients should have compatible blood types and an emotional bond. Unlike other transplants, livers do not need to be matched by tissue type. The donor liver, however, must be of sufficient size that a lobe will be large enough for the recipient.

The living donor undergoes careful medical, psychological, and social evaluation. Potential donors may be rejected because their livers are unsuitable or they have underlying medical conditions that increase the risk of complications from surgery.

Risk to the donor is small but present. The current estimate of the risk of death is 1 in 500 liver donations. Other complications can occur, however, including pulmonary emboli, gastrointestinal bleeding, bile duct injury, bile leak, and infection. The overall rate of serious complications in donors is approximately 10 percent. The liver is the only internal human organ that regenerates itself; the portion of the liver that is removed regenerates over 8 to 16 weeks.

The overall outcome for recipients primarily relates to their pre-transplant clinical condition. When the procedure is performed in stable patients under non-urgent conditions, the one-year survival rate is greater than 90 percent. Survival rates decrease when the transplant takes place in more urgent circumstances. It is likely that living-donor liver transplantation will become commonplace in the future, and selection criteria will change.

The NIH recently funded a multicenter study to carefully examine performance and outcome of liver donor liver transplantation in the United States. The clinical centers participating in this study include:

- *University of Colorado, Denver*
- *University of California, San Francisco*
- *University of California, Los Angeles*
- *Virginian Commonwealth University, Richmond*
- *Columbia—Cornell University, New York*
- *University of Virginia, Charlottesville*
- *University of North Carolina, Chapel Hill*

THE SURGICAL PROCEDURE. The human body has two kidneys, two lungs—but only one liver. Scientists have created artificial kidneys (kidney dialysis) and even artificial hearts, but no one has been able to duplicate the hundreds of functions of the liver to create an effective liver dialysis machine. Liver transplant surgery, therefore, has no fallback position, no margin for error.

Although the original method pioneered by Dr. Starzl has been modified, the basic technique remains essentially unchanged. The operation has three phases:

1. *Dissection to access the patient's liver*
2. *Removal of the patient's liver*
3. *Connecting the donated liver*

First, the surgeon meticulously dissects tissues and promptly controls bleeding vessels to expose the patient's liver. This process takes about one to two hours. Blood loss ranges from zero to 5 pints of red blood cells.

In the next phase, the surgeon clamps the blood vessels supplying your liver and removes the liver. Then the surgeon and anesthesiologist work together to maintain adequate blood clotting factors. The anesthesiologist carefully monitors your blood and blood pressure to give you the proper fluids and blood products. In the last phase, the surgeon positions the donor liver in your abdomen and sews the blood vessels together. This procedure takes from one-and-one-half to three hours; blood loss ranges from zero to 5 pints.

Once all the vessels are connected, the surgeon must unclamp the main vessels. After unclamping, one of the more critical periods of the procedure begins—especially if your blood clotting is poor. After you stabilize, your surgeon connects your bile duct to the donor bile duct and removes the donor gallbladder.

Livers typically begin to function immediately after their blood supply is established. Clotting improves, and the liver makes bile on the operating table.

"The most critical moment in the operation," says University of Colorado's Chief of Transplantation, Dr. Igal Kam, "is when we release the clamps holding the vessels going to the new liver, and the new liver changes in color from pale or dark brown to a more pink-brown, because new blood is flowing to the liver. When we see the yellow-brown bile start to appear from the bile duct, we can relax because we know the liver is going to work. There's no room for mistakes in this procedure.

"About 40 to 50 percent of patients go off the respirator in the operating room and we can talk to them. After six to eight hours of surgery, it's great to talk to the patient. We deal with very sick people who sometimes have only hours to live. After the transplant, then we see the miracle."

THE HOSPITAL STAY.   After the operation you may be monitored in an intensive care unit (ICU) where the staff is specifically trained to manage this early post-transplant period. Patients who are very stable may bypass the ICU and transfer from recovery room directly to the transplant inpatient floor. If you are transferred to the ICU and have no complications, you'll spend 24 to 48 hours in the ICU and then transfer to the inpatient transplant unit.

Usually, patients stay in the hospital from five to 20 days depending on their condition. Some people require extensive rehabilitation, such as physical therapy or nursing, due to their weakened situation before the transplant.

The operation was a corker. I was on the table for eight to nine hours and had several transfusions. I lost a lot of blood.

When I was in a post-operative coma, it was weird. I was asking my brother if I was in the C.I.A. I told him, "You've got to get me out of here. They're trying to bump me off." I had all kinds of weird dreams.

The transplant went real well. I was in the hospital for five days. I was fighting to get out because Thanksgiving was coming up, and my son was coming to visit.
The TV sucked—three to four channels, no cable. The food wasn't much better. On Thanksgiving morning, the whole medical crew came in, and the nurse asked if I could go home, because my son was coming from college. I was released that day.

After discharge you'll be monitored in transplant outpatient clinics for a few weeks to a few months, and then you'll return to the care of your referring primary care physician or gastroenterologist. The transplant center continues to guide patient management through close cooperation with referring physicians.

Living with a New Liver

Although highly variable from patient to patient, most people require from three to six months to physically recover from surgery and adjust to new medications. An inspiration to transplant athletes, Chris Klug, a 28-year-old American snowboarder, took the gold in the World Cup parallel giant slalom on January 17, 2001—less than nine months after his liver transplant for primary sclerosing cholangitis.

Liver transplantation is a profound event that affects every part of a patient's life—the mind as well as the body. Patients must learn to live with lifelong medications, deal with the fear of rejection of the organ, and come to terms with a profound physical and psychological transformation.

MEDICATIONS TO PREVENT REJECTION. After the transplant, you need to take medications for the rest of your life to prevent your immune system from rejecting your new liver. The medications are called immunosuppressants and include the following: cyclosporine (Sandimmune, Neoral), tacrolimus (Prograf), sirolimus (Rapamune) azathioprine (Imuran), steroids (Prednisone, Solumedrol), and mycophenolate mofetil (Cellcept).

I took four different meds the first week. They had a grid set up as to when I took what. They had me on Prograf, a high dose—8 milligrams. I was on 5 milligrams for a while. Then they cut me to 4 milligrams a day.

The first two weeks after my transplant, I had a slight rejection. They take you down and give you an I.V. treatment. They did that twice within the first two or three weeks, and that was it.

I called OKT3 rocket fuel during my stay on it. It whacked me out.

In 1993, I started having heart palpitations, and I was fatigued all the time. They did a biopsy and found that all that was left functioning of my liver was 10 to 15 percent. I had over a pound of iron in my liver.

My first transplant was pretty rough going. I had different rejection episodes before things straightened out. My iron stores were normal for about a year and a half. Then I had a couple of phlebotomies, but a bad infection put an end to that for about five years. Then I got sick again and got tired easily.

They diagnosed me with a clotted hepatic artery. Blood wasn't getting to the bile ducts. First they opened the blockages, which worked for a while. Then they put tubes down the bile duct to drain bile through a hole in my ribcage. Two bags hung off my side in a holster under my clothes.

I was fading fast and was put back on the transplant list for one day before I got the call that they had a donor.

Most patients take either cyclosporine, tacrolimus, or sirolimus as primary therapy, and use the other agents to strengthen the anti-rejection effect. In the first six to twelve months it's common to take two or three anti-rejection medications. After that period most patients remain on cyclosporine, tacrolimus, or sirolimus, either alone or in combination with low-dose Prednisone.

Although the medications have side effects, most of them are dose-related and respond to either lowering the dose of the specific immunosuppressant or changing to another medication.

Never change doses by yourself. All dose adjustments of immunosuppressants require the supervision of your doctor. If you take too little immunosuppression, you run the risk of rejecting your liver transplant. If you take too much immunosuppression, you risk infection, renal (kidney) failure, hypertension, hyperlipidemia (excess blood cholesterol and fat), and diabetes mellitus.

MANAGING COMPLICATIONS. It's essential that your transplant team supervise you closely during your post-transplant outpatient care. The most concerning problem for patients with hemochromatosis is rejection.

REJECTION. If rejection occurs, it typically does so within the first three months of the transplant and is detected by a rise in liver enzymes. Elevations of liver enzymes and bilirubin occur, although the first change noted is usually an increase in AST. In some cases, rejection is very mild and does not require additional immunosuppressive treatment. In more severe cases of rejection, the patient may experience fever (up to 102°F), poor appetite, fatigue, and malaise.

Nearly all rejections occur within three months of transplantation, but occasionally rejection happens later. "Late rejection" usually results from low levels of immunosuppressive therapy due to improper dosing, addition of a new medication, or development of a simultaneous illness such as diarrhea or liver dysfunction. Rejection usually responds to intravenous steroids or other strategies (OKT3).

INFECTION. The early postoperative period is the time of greatest risk for infection. The most common infections during this period are bacterial and related to the operation, wound, and catheters. It is common to experience thrush (yeast infection of the mouth) or fever blisters (herpetic outbreak of the lips), but these respond quickly to medications. Rarely, more serious viral or fungal infections can occur and require prolonged hospitalization and specialized treatments.

Although the period of greatest risk is early post-transplant, lifetime use of immunosuppression increases your chances for infection even in the long run. Monitor your condition closely and immediately report new symptoms, especially fever, chills, night sweats, loss of appetite, and weight loss, to your physician. A search for underlying infection may be warranted.

SIDE EFFECTS OF MEDICATIONS. A number of side effects can occur with the currently used immunosuppressive medications. Here are some of the more common ones:

CYCLOSPORINE	HIGH BLOOD PRESSURE
	HIGH CHOLESTEROL AND TRIGLYCERIDE
	KIDNEY DYSFUNCTION
	WEIGHT GAIN
	GOUT
	GROWTH IN BODY HAIR
TACROLIMUS	KIDNEY DYSFUNCTION
	GOUT
	NUMBNESS, TINGLING OF EXTREMITIES
	DIABETES
PREDNISONE	HIGH BLOOD PRESSURE
	HIGH CHOLESTEROL AND TRIGLYCERIDE
	OBESITY
	DIABETES
MYCOPHENOLATE	LOW WHITE BLOOD COUNT
	GASTROINTESTINAL UPSET, DIARRHEA
SIROLIMUS (RAPAMYCIN)	MOUTH SORES
	LOW WHITE BLOOD COUNT

After the transplant, your physicans and nurses monitor you for development of any of these side effects. When they occur, you might require changes in the dosing of your immunosuppressive prescription, conversion to a different immunosuppressive medication, or addition of another type of medication to combat the side effect. For example, you might need anti-hypertensive medications to treat high blood pressure due to the immunosuppressive medications.

PSYCHOLOGICAL TRANSFORMATION. Post-transplant patients go through a period of accepting the "gift of life." The feelings are common to everyone and include curiosity about the donor, feelings of guilt that someone had to die so they could live, and a sense of indebtedness—of feeling overwhelmed and struggling with how to repay an enormous gift.

>   When I first found out I had HH, I was in the intensive care unit. The doctor said, "I don't know if I can save your life." My wife cried. It was a roller coaster, nerve-wracking—with phlebotomies and GI scopes. I retreated into myself.
>   At first, I thought, "What am I going to do? Well, hell, if I have to die, then I'll die. And that's the way it is. I kind of accepted it.
>   I deal with stuff internally and kind of forget about others around me. But my wife is younger, and it's hard on her.

I had to leave college, but I went back to finish when I got back on my feet after the transplant. It took two years to get back on my feet.

Hindsight is 20/20. I was somewhat naïve. I knew I was sick, but I never considered that there wouldn't be a liver for me. I never thought I'd die—and that sustained me. But with hindsight, I was very close to passing away before I got my liver.

There's got to be some reason I made it. Transplantation is a difficult business. What's the reality? Two to three people die waiting for a liver.

You're given a hand, and you have to deal with it. It opens your eyes and gives you a feeling of compassion, of caring for other people.

If people think they can't do something, I'm living proof that you can. I went back to school at age 50 after a liver transplant. I was disabled. Now I've retrained in computer networking. I've got a car, a townhome.

I went to the transplant games in 1996, 1998, and 2000 in Florida. They're just like the regular Olympics. I competed in golf and table tennis. Can't do track because of arthritis.

Four years after the operation, I built another house for myself. I'm a fireman and active in my church. People have a hard time believing that I had a liver transplant until I pick up my shirt and show them the scar.

I wrote letters to both donors, but I still haven't heard from either one. It's up to them to answer or not. Sometimes people need time to get over things before they can get things out in the open.

Thank God for donors and for transplantation.

Michael Talamantes, transplant social worker at the University of Colorado Health Sciences Center, says that patients often write a letter of thanks to the donor's family. The donor's identity is kept confidential, so the letter is sent through official channels. If the donor's family members wish to reply, they will. And if not, it's important to respect their privacy.

Feelings of guilt over the donor's death take time to work through. Although it seems obvious that the donor's death is independent of your need for a liver, the feelings are almost universal.

The sense of indebtedness is often overwhelming. Some people do community service or visit patients in the hospital who are awaiting transplants. Every patient is touched in some way.

As in every new experience, you may have contradictory feelings. It's important to pay attention to them. Whatever normal, contradictory feelings you have, you need to sort through them to adjust to your new sense of yourself. To complicate matters, you may get mixed messages from others. Are you a hero, a biotechnological miracle, or does your boss see you as damaged goods, a drain on the company's health insurance? Whatever your experiences, they are profound indeed. You are not alone in wrestling with these issues.

Improved Survival Rates

OVERALL OUTCOME AFTER LIVER TRANSPLANTATION. The heartening news is that survival rates have increased due to advances in immunosuppression (beginning with cyclosporine in 1979) and the team approach to liver transplantation. Before cyclosporine, patients were treated with high doses of prednisone and azathioprine. Procedures, such as thoracic duct drainage, splenectomy, and anti-lymphocyte immunoglobulin injections, were used to further suppress the immune system and prevent rejection. Before 1979, results were poor: 32 percent of patients survived one year and only 22 percent survived 30 months.

The picture has changed dramatically. Liver transplant results show that average one-, three-, and five-year patient survival rates in patients transplanted between 1988 and 1997 are 82 percent, 75 percent, and 71 percent. Similar results are being reported from Europe and Asia. Results from individual centers are even more impressive with many reporting one-year patient survivals in excess of 90 percent.

OUTCOME IN PATIENTS WITH HEMOCHROMATOSIS. Many, perhaps the majority of people with HH, do extremely well with little evidence of significant damage over years of follow-up. However, some patients with extensive iron overload experience complications, and even death, related to cardiac compromise and infection in the postoperative period.

Several reports have suggested that post-transplant survival of HH patients is reduced compared to controls.

	HH	CONTROL
STUDY 1: ONE YEAR SURVIVAL	58%	79%
STUDY 2: ONE YEAR SURVIVAL	54%	79%
FIVE YEAR SURVIVAL	43%	69%
STUDY 3: ONE YEAR SURVIVAL	52%	80%

None of these reports tested for HFE mutations. The diagnosis of hemochromatosis was based upon clinical, biochemical and histological data.

A recent study from the Mayo Clinic examined not only the impact of iron overload but also HFE mutation. The five year survival after liver transplant in patients with hepatic iron overload (HII > 1.9) of 48 percent was significantly lower than the five year survival of 77 percent for controls without iron overload (Figure 11A). However, most of the patients represented by this data had iron overload that was unrelated to HFE mutations. Only 4 of 41 patients with iron overload had C282Y homozygosity (10 percent). There were no compound heterozygotes. Although 7 had C282Y heterozygosity (18 percent), and 9 had H63D heterozygosity (23 percent), these mutations are not typically associated with iron overload.

Thus, approximately 90 percent of patients with hepatic iron overload who have end-stage cirrhosis and undergo liver transplantation lack the classic HFE mutations. They have iron overload due to other causes. The implication is that iron overload, not HFE mutations per se, increases the risk of serious complications after liver transplantation.

The reality is, however, that not all patients survive after liver transplantation. Deaths occurring within the first six months are due to non-function of the donor's liver, clotting of the main artery to the liver, infection, multi-organ failure, or rejection. When deaths occur later after the transplant, they are more commonly due to malignancy or complications of atherosclerosis, rejection, or infection.

Patients with hemochromatosis or iron overload may be particularly prone to infectious complications after liver transplantation. In one study, infection-related deaths, particularly due to fungus, were much more common in patients with iron overload (24 percent vs. 7 percent).

FIGURE 11. IRON OVERLOAD IN CIRRHOSIS—HFE GENOTYPES AND OUTCOME AFTER LIVER TRANSPLANTATION

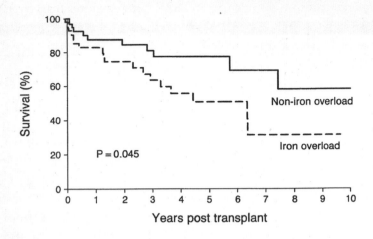

The outlook is very hopeful. We anticipate that current immunosuppressive protocols will reduce adverse metabolic effects and continue to improve the long-term outlook for transplant recipients. Our ultimate goal, of course, is to restore you to your normal life.

Issues in Liver Transplantation for the Carrier (C282Y Heterozygote)

A recent paper addressed three issues in liver transplantation relevant to the C282Y carrier:

First, heterozygotes are not more likely to undergo liver transplantation than the general population. The prevalence of C282Y heterozygosity was 8.6 percent in 304 recipients of liver transplantation, compared to a prevalence of 8.4 percent in a group of 5211 volunteer blood donors. If heterozygosity to C282Y increased the likelihood of liver failure, liver cancer, and the need for liver transplantation, one would expect an increased prevalence of C282Y in transplant recipients.

Second, heterozygotes had the same post-transplant survival and outcome as transplant recipients without C282Y.

Third, organs from donors carrying one mutation of C282Y have the same post-transplant outcome as organs from donors negative for C282Y. Twenty-four C282Y heterozygotes were detected in a pool of 141 donors. Graft and recipient survival of those who received the

C282Y grafts was identical to graft and recipient survival of those who received unaffected grafts.

In general this is good news for C282Y heterozygotes (carriers). You are not at increased risk to get a liver transplant. If you do need a transplant for another reason, such as hepatitis C, then your post-transplant outcome is not worsened because you are a carrier. In addition, should you elect to be an organ donor (either cadaveric or living) then your graft will function properly in a recipient.

How Organs Are Allocated

UNOS. In the United States, the United Network for Organ-Sharing (UNOS) regulates the distribution or allocation of donor organs. Here's how it works.

The United States is divided into 11 regions for organ procurement and allocation. Several local organ procurement organizations (OPOs) exist within each region. When a patient is approved for transplantation, he or she is placed on local, regional, and national waiting lists. Typically, more than 80 percent of recipients receive organs from local donors.

LISTING STATUS. A patient placed on the waiting list is given a UNOS status, or priority, based upon severity of disease. UNOS 1 is the most urgent status. Patients in this category have acute irreversible liver failure and are not likely to survive beyond seven days without transplantation. MELD (Model for End-stage Liver Disease) score has essentially replaced the other UNOS listing categories (2A, 2B, 3). MELD score is calculated from bilirubin, prothrombin time, and creatinine, and listing scores range from 6 (lowest priority) to 40 (highest priority). MELD score predicts short-term (three-month) survival; those with the highest MELD score are least likely to survive three months and have the most urgent need for transplantation.

As the waiting list continues to expand, will a shortage of donors lead to increasing numbers of people dying while they wait for a liver? The number of patients listed more than quintupled from 1988 to 1998, but the number of liver transplants only doubled. In 1988, 214 patients on the waiting list died. In 1994, 694 patients died, and in 2000, 1636 died. As a society we need to find solutions to the organ shortage.

CENTERS OF EXCELLENCE. UNOS displays the results for liver transplantation in the United States on its continually updated Web site, www.unos.org. Patient and graft survivals for one- and three-year outcomes are given in combined totals and for each individual center. Results are also adjusted for differences in patient populations according to variables known to influence outcome after liver transplantation: UNOS listing status, diagnosis of fulminant hepatic failure, age, renal failure, presence of hepatitis B, and presence of primary liver cancer. Using this stratification method, results from each center can be compared to the expected outcome. Intuitively, one could suggest that this analysis identifies true "centers of excellence," because it is based solely upon adjusted medical outcomes.

Medicare was the first to put into practice the concept of centers of excellence in liver transplantation. Additional third-party insurers, such as Blue Cross/Blue Shield, Prudential, United Resource Network, and Kaiser Permanente use similar criteria. With the explosion of HMOs the criteria for designating centers of excellence are more a mixture of medical outcome and economic impact. Adoption of standardized medical criteria for designation of "centers of excellence" would eliminate the potential that a given program could be an insurer's transplant center by simply offering the lowest price

Many people have suggested that the current number of 117 transplant programs is far in excess of what the donor organ pool can provide. More than half the programs in the U.S. perform fewer than 20 liver transplants per year; 75 percent of all liver transplants are performed by only 25 percent of the programs.

A recent publication by UNOS in *The New England Journal of Medicine* indicated that transplant teams that perform more than 20 transplants per year achieve optimal patient and graft survival. According to this analysis, the chance to die after liver transplantation is almost twice as great when the transplant is done by a program performing fewer than 20 transplants per year. Because more than half the programs in the U.S. perform fewer than 20 transplants a year, one must question the wisdom of encouraging the proliferation of transplant centers.

RESOURCE: Call the toll-free UNOS patient information number at 1-888-TXINFO1 (1-888-894-6361); Web site: www.unos.org. To request free single copies of the following brochures, write to UNOS, P.O. Box 2484, Richmond, VA 23218: *What Every Patient Needs to Know; Share Your Life. Share Your Decision.*

RESOURCE: Updated waitlist and transplant summary reports, statistics by state, region, or individual hospitals, and other information are available on the UNOS Web site: www.unos.org.

RESOURCE: Regional organ recovery organizations are a good source of information. To locate your region's organization, call the UNOS patient information number listed above.

RESOURCE: For information on national organizations and local coalitions that educate the public about organ donation, call the Coalition on Donation: 804-782-4920. Email: coalition@shareyourlife.org; Web site: www.shareyourlife.org.

RESOURCE: For a free Transplant Support Group Directory of pre- and post-transplant support groups nationwide, call Chronimed Pharmacy: 1-800-888-5753 and ask for a patient specialist.

RESOURCE: For information about transplants and organ donation, call a nationwide support group for transplant patients and their families, Transplant Recipients International Organization (TRIO): 1-800-TRIO-386.

RESOURCE: A uniform donor card is enclosed in this book. Discuss organ and tissue donation with family members. After completing and signing the Uniform Donor Card, be sure to have your signature witnessed by two people.

Stone walls do not a prison make,
Nor iron bars a cage;
RICHARD LOVELACE

12

RESEARCH TRENDS

Hope for the Future

My feeling is that some day we'll have a pill to remove iron. That would sure beat phlebotomy treatments. If people can take a pill for high cholesterol, why can't researchers develop one for iron?

KEVIN

S A HEPATOLOGIST WHO EVALUATES AND advises patients with hemochromatosis, I have observed great improvements in our understanding, detection, and treatment of this condition. However, even today many patients escape early detection and develop advanced liver disease or other organ dysfunction from iron overload. Nonetheless, research into appropriate screening methods is advancing, and our understanding of the mechanisms of iron absorption continues to leap forward. I look with anticipation toward the next few years, and I expect to see exciting new advances.

Hemochromatosis research falls into two broad and somewhat overlapping categories: clinical research and basic research. Clinical research primarily determines whether new screening strategies or therapeutic interventions are effective. Basic research encompasses a wide variety of studies of hemochromatosis, including, but not limited to molecular biology, cell biology, transplantation, pathophysiology, and pharmacology.

In this final chapter, we'll cover the following topics:

- *Clinical Research*
    RELATIONSHIP BETWEEN GENOTYPE AND PHENOTYPE
    OPTIMAL SCREENING PROCEDURES
    COST-EFFECTIVENESS OF SCREENING
    ETHICAL, LEGAL AND SOCIAL IMPLICATIONS OF SCREENING
- *Role As a Study Subject in Clinical Research*
- *Basic Research*
    UNDERSTANDING THE STEPS THAT LEAD TO IRON
        OVERLOAD
    ANIMAL AND CELL CULTURE MODELS.
- *Summary*

Clinical Research

RELATIONSHIP BETWEEN GENOTYPE AND PHENOTYPE (CLINICAL EXPRESSION). Several studies have begun to examine the relationship of HFE mutations to the level of iron overload and organ damage. Risk factors for disease progression are under investigation, including the impact of age, gender, ethnicity, alcohol, smoking, and coincident liver disease. A number of recent publications throughout the world testify to the interest in defining the impact of genotype on tissue accumulation of iron, organ damage, and clinical expression of disease. Future studies will confirm results and establish greater understanding of the complex relationships between genetic makeup and clinical disease. In addition, risk factors for disease progression will be defined.

OPTIMAL SCREENING PROCEDURES. Principles of screening populations for a given disease or condition were defined by Wilson and Jungner in 1968. These principles included the following:

- *The condition must be important to the public health.*
- *There must be an accurate screening test.*
- *There should be effective treatment that could be administered during the early, silent stages and prevent emergence of disease.*
- *The cost of screening must be offset by benefits to the patient that maintain health, enhance productivity, and sustain quality of life.*

One could argue that hemochromatosis is a condition that satisfies all of the above criteria for screening. It is a common condition, accurate screening methods exist (HFE mutations), phlebotomy is effective therapy, and cost of treatment is relatively small when one considers the potential costs of disease progression in untreated patients. Potential costs of disease progression encompass costs related to liver disease and cirrhosis (outpatient visits, procedures, hospitalizations, TIPS), hospitalizations due to complications, treatments of liver failure and liver cancer, and transplantation.

However, genetic screening of the population has not yet been recommended for these reasons:

- *Uncertainty of natural history.*
- *Age-related expression of disease.*
- *Optimal management of the asymptomatic patient.*
- *Psychological impact of genetic testing.*
- *Cost (approximately $110,000 per detected case of homozygous C282Y).*

One study screened 41,038 individuals attending a U.S. health appraisal clinic and found 152 C282Y homozygotes. Only one of the 152 homozygotes had symptoms and signs to suggest hemochromatosis. These results point out two key features of hemochromatosis. First, many patients have a relatively benign course and prolonged asymptomatic period. On the other hand, the only sure way to reliably detect the asymptomatic early period of hemochromatosis is by genetic testing.

Nonetheless, many investigators have raised concerns about identifying and treating patients when they are asymptomatic. Current research is focusing on the medical, psychological, legal and ethical issues surrounding population genetic testing. Several future and ongoing studies will begin to define:

- *Natural history, particularly age-related disease expression;*
- *Nature and prevalence of HFE mutations in specific ethnic or cultural groups;*
- *New HFE and non-HFE mutations associated with iron overload;*
- *Morbidity associated with HFE mutations;*
- *Mortality associated with HFE mutations;*
- *Benefits of early treatment.*

COST-EFFECTIVENESS OF SCREENING. The costs of screening must be balanced by the chance to detect hemochromatosis at an early stage and prevent clinical disease. Suggested screening strategies range from genetic screening of the entire population to selected use of genetic tests only in those with iron overload or who are first-degree relatives of a C282Y homozygote. Research into screening strategies relies heavily on models with a number of assumptions that are based upon reported studies and best estimates.

The most established screening methods for hemochromatosis employ tests that measure excess iron, such as transferrin saturation. This test costs approximately $12. The cost to detect one case of homozygous C282Y is approximately $2,700. The unbound iron binding capacity is less costly ($1), but its operating characteristics are less well defined than transferrin saturation.

Although these tests are effective in detecting 92 percent of affected family members in pedigree studies, they are much less sensitive when applied to studies of larger, general populations. For example, screening of blood donors with transferrin saturation may detect less than 50 percent of patients with C282Y homozygosity. The use of genetic tests as screening tools is gaining interest, because they are more sensitive and would detect virtually detect all C282Y homozygotes. So, why not abandon iron-based screening and move entirely towards genetic screening?

Let's look at some of the issues regarding genetic screening of the whole U.S. population. Screening would probably be limited to that portion of the population that is of European descent, or approximately 200,000,000 persons. Approximately 1 in 200, or 1,000,000 persons, would be homozygous for C282Y mutation and at risk for HFE-related hemochromatosis. If the lifetime risk for development of organ damage, organ dysfunction, or death related to hemochromatosis is approximately 20 percent, then only 200,000 individuals would benefit from detection and institution of treatment. If the cost of the gene tests were approximately $200, then 40 billion dollars would be spent on screening alone.

However, detection of affected individuals incurs additional costs. Once a C282Y homozygote was detected, additional testing to define iron overload would be necessary. Some people would need a liver biopsy, and some would require extensive medical or even surgical treatments.

Given these variables and others, Adams has suggested that the cost of genetic tests currently prohibits their use in screening strategies. However, Adams also indicated that if costs of genetic tests decreased to $28, screening with gene testing could become the most effective strategy. Obviously, additional research is needed in this controversial and important area of clinical investigation.

ETHICAL, LEGAL, AND SOCIAL IMPLICATIONS OF SCREENING. Several issues of potential discrimination are raised by the specter of genetic testing. If you are a child or adolescent and test positive for C282Y, will you be denied insurance when you reach adult age? Or, will you only be able to purchase insurance that excludes coverage for illness related to liver disease, heart disease, or diabetes? Similar questions arise in the minds of adults considering testing.

Employers might avoid hiring a person who may be susceptible to disease, require sick leave, sustain hospitalizations, and increase premium rates on group health plans. In this regard, results of genetic tests could form the basis for genetic discrimination in the workplace.

Results of genetic tests might change one's perception of self and influence interactions with family friends and loved ones.

Several areas for research have been identified:

- *Insurance of privacy in the use and interpretation of genetic tests;*
- *Methods of counseling affected persons and family members;*
- *Process and adequacy of informed consent for screening;*
- *Development of public and professional education programs.*

Role as a Study Subject in Clinical Research

Should you sign up for a study? Obviously, before you enroll in a specific study, you should take time to review the patient informed consent document that you will have to sign. Be sure to ask how often you will see a doctor; doctor appointments vary at different study sites. You should also consider all the pros and cons of any study.

On the positive side:

1. In treatment trials, you may get to try a new treatment that is not available through general clinical practice.

2. Typically, you would receive frequent examinations and careful follow-up.

3. Study coordinators will keep you informed about your status and progress.

4. Most studies are sponsored by research grants, and typically your treatment is delivered without expense to you or your insurer. However, the degree of compensation can vary and you (or your insurer) may be responsible for some of the bill. Some studies also give extra compensation to you for expenses related to travel to the study site or for the time you spent participating in the research.

5. Your participation is kept confidential. Representatives from the FDA or study sponsors, however, have the right to review your study record.

6. You reserve the right to stop treatment and withdraw from the study at any time.

On the negative side:

1. Testing programs are rigid. You must make the time commitment to follow the protocol exactly. For example, you'll have to show up at certain times for follow-up tests.

2. Clinical trials of medications are usually blinded. If you agree to participate in this type of trial, you won't know what you're getting in terms of dosage or placebo, for example. If you have been given a placebo, the sponsor may offer the active treatment to you (free of charge) at the end of your participation in the trial if you completed the study. However, the sponsor is under no obligation to do this.

3. Sponsors can stop the trials at any time.

4. You may experience undocumented side effects.

5. You must be prepared to reveal all aspects of your physical and emotional health.

6. You won't know the results of the whole study, or your individual results, until every participant has completed the protocol. It may take more than a year from your point of enrollment.

> RESOURCE: Many organizations listed in the Resources section at the back of this book offer information about research studies. In addition, the National Institutes of Health (NIH) supplies descriptions of current HH studies and enrollment information. Web site: ClinicalTrials.gov

Basic Research

A review by Philpott recently identified eight areas of basic investigation into the mechanism of iron overload in hemochromatosis:

- *Iron uptake in the intestinal lining cells;*

- ◆ *Transfer of iron from the intestinal cell into blood;*
- ◆ *Uptake of iron by cells within the body;*
- ◆ *Control mechanisms for intestinal iron uptake;*
- ◆ *Role of HFE in control of intestinal iron uptake;*
- ◆ *Interactions between specific proteins and iron;*
- ◆ *Role of newly discovered proteins, such as Hepcidin;*
- ◆ *Models for the control of absorption of dietary iron.*

UNDERSTANDING THE STEPS THAT LEAD TO IRON OVERLOAD. Let's reexamine some of the steps involved in iron absorption by the intestinal lining cells and delivery of the iron to the various cells of the body. Dietary iron is in an oxidized state (ferric). It must be reduced to its ferrous form prior to absorption by the cell. A specific ferrireductase protein (Dcytb) in the surface of the intestinal lining cells converts ferric to ferrous iron. Ferrous iron is then transported across the plasma membrane of the intestinal lining cell via another specific protein (DMT1). Iron leaves the intestinal lining cell to gain entry into the blood compartment via another specific protein, ferroportin 1 (FP1). Circulating iron is typically bound to transferrin and enters the cells of the body after transferrin binds to its specfic receptor, the transferrin receptor.

The control of iron uptake is undoubtedly quite complex, and great strides in understanding have been achieved through studies in animals, cell culture, and humans. Future research studies are needed to further define the regulation and mechanisms of control of the activity of:

- ◆ *Ferrireductase (Dcytb);*
- ◆ *DMT1;*
- ◆ *Ferroportin 1 (FP1);*
- ◆ *Transferrin and transferrin receptor;*
- ◆ *HFE;*
- ◆ *Hepcidin.*

ANIMAL AND CELL CULTURE MODELS. Until recently, studies of hemochromatosis have been hampered by lack of a convenient experimental model. The ideal model for studying hemochromatosis would be one that mimics the condition in humans and is affordable, widely available, and allows for easily reproducible manipulation of experimental conditions. Several mouse (HFE -/-, hpx, mk) and cell culture models (HeLa cells, Chinese hamster ovary cells, macrophages, red cells) that mimic certain aspects of human hemochromatosis are currently used in studies of molecular mechanisms of iron overload.

Summary

It is my hope that we are entering a new era in the understanding of hemochromatosis, in which research may ultimately lead to discoveries of more effective treatments that benefit patients. For example, one could envision medications that inhibit iron absorption by selectively regulating specific proteins or their genes in the intestinal lining cells. The development of such a therapeutic strategy could theoretically limit or eliminate the need for phlebotomy.

Research into the basic mechanisms of hemochromatosis is absolutely essential so that our understanding and treatment of this condition may leap forward. Clearly, research that results in better treatment ultimately saves money as well as lives. Hemochromatosis patients, friends, and family members must focus attention on research. We must make it a priority to confront, define, and treat hereditary hemochromatosis.

Iron rusts from disuse; stagnant water loses its purity and in cold weather becomes frozen; even so does inaction sap the vigor of the mind.
LEONARDO DA VINCI

RESOURCES

Hemochromatosis Organizations

AMERICAN HEMOCHROMATOSIS SOCIETY, INC.
4044 W. Lake Mary Blvd., #104, PMB 416
Lake Mary, FL 32746-2012
Toll-Free Information Hotline: 1-888-655-IRON (4766)
Office: 407-829-4488
Web site: www.americanhs.org
Email: mail@americanhs.org

THE CANADIAN HEMOCHROMATOSIS SOCIETY
272-7000 Minoru Blvd.
Richmond, B.C.
Canada V6Y 3Z5
Toll-Free in Canada (outside Vancouver and Lower Mainland):
1-877-BAD-IRON (223-4766)
Office: 604-279-7135
Web site: www/cdnhemochromatosis.ca
Email: office@cdnhemochromatosis.ca

HEMOCHROMATOSIS FOUNDATION, INC.
P.O. Box 8569
Albany, NY 12208-0569
518-489-0972
Web site: www.hemochromatosis.org
Email: s.kleiner@shiva.hunter.cuny.edu

IRON DISORDERS INSTITUTE, INC.
P.O. Box 2031
Greenville, SC 29602
Toll-Free National Information Request Line: 1-888-565-IRON (4766)
864-292-1175
Web site: www.irondisorders.org
Email: irondis@aol.com

IRON OVERLOAD DISEASES ASSOCIATION, INC.
433 Westwind Drive
North Palm Beach, FL 33408
561-840-8512
561-840-8513
Web site: www.ironoverload.org
Email: iod@ironoverload.org

Other Organizations

AMERICAN DIABETES ASSOCIATION
Attn: National Call Center
1701 N. Beauregard St.
Alexandria, VA 22311
Toll-Free: 1-800-DIABETES (1-800-342-2383)
Web site: www.diabetes.org
Email: AskADA@diabetes.org

AMERICAN HEART ASSOCIATION NATIONAL CENTER
7272 Greenville Ave.
Dallas, TX 75231
Toll-Free: 1-800-AHA-USA-1 (242-8721)
Web site: www.americanheart.org

AMERICAN LIVER FOUNDATION
75 Maiden Lane, Suite 603
New York, NY 10038
Toll-Free: 1-800-GO-LIVER (465-4837); 1-888-443-7222
212-668-1000
Web site: www.liverfoundation.org
Email: info@liverfoundation.org

ARTHRITIS FOUNDATION
P.O. Box 7669
Atlanta, GA 30357-0669
Toll-Free: 1-800-283-7800
Web site: www.arthritis.org

GENETIC ALLIANCE
4301 Connecticut Avenue, N.W.
Suite 404
Washington, D.C. 20008-2304
202-966-5557
Toll-Free Helpline: 1-800-336-GENE
Web site: www.geneticalliance.org
Email: info@geneticalliance.org

NATIONAL ASSOCIATION FOR RARE DISORDERS, INC.
55 Kenosia Ave.
P.O. Box 1968
Danbury, CT 06813-1968
Toll-Free: 1-800-999-6673 (voicemail)
TDD: 203-797-9590
203-744-0100
Web site: www.rarediseases.org
Email: orphan@rarediseases.org

NATIONAL SOCIETY OF GENETIC COUNSELORS, INC.
233 Canterbury Drive
Wallingford, PA 19086
610-872-7608
Web site: www.nsgc.org
Email: nsgc@nsgc.org

Government Agencies

CENTERS FOR DISEASE CONTROL AND PREVENTION (CDC)
Division of Nutrition and Physical Activity
Office of Genetics and Disease Prevention
For Public Inquiries:
Centers for Disease Control and Prevention
Public Inquiries/MASO
Mailstop F07
1600 Clifton Rd.
Atlanta, GA 30333
Public Inquiries: 404-639-3534; Toll-Free: 1-800-311-3435
404-639-3311
Web site: www.cdc.gov
Email: Access Web site, "Contact Us"

THE **NATIONAL INSTITUTES OF HEALTH (NIH)** is the largest bio-medical research center in the world. It's the research arm of the Public Health Service, U.S. Department of Health and Human Services. NIH Visitor Information Center: 301-496-1776; www.nih.gov.
The NIH offers reliable and helpful resources, including the following:
National Institute of Diabetes & Digestive & Kidney Diseases (NIDDK)
National Digestive Diseases Information Clearinghouse (NDDIC)
2 Information Way
Bethesda, MD 20892-3570
Web site: www.niddk.nih.gov
Email: nddic@info.niddk.nih.gov

CHID Online (Combined Health Information Database):
www.chid.nih.gov
The National Library of Medicine in collaboration with the NIH:
www.medlineplus.gov
The National Human Genome Research Institute leads the Human Genome Project for the NIH. Its Web site provides information on genetic research, health, and policy and ethics: www.genome.gov.
The Genetic and Rare Diseases Information Center (supported by the Office of Rare Diseases and the National Human Genome Research Institute, both of the NIH):
Office of Rare Diseases
National Institutes of Health
6100 Executive Boulevard,
Room 3A07, MSC 7518
Bethesda, Maryland 20892-7518
301-402-4336
Genetic and Rare Diseases Information Center: 1-888-205-2311
    (TTY) 1-888-205-3223
Email: ord@od.nih.gov
Web site: http://rarediseases.info.nih.gov (Click on
    "Genetic Information.")

Transplant Organizations and Agencies

TRANSPLANT RECIPIENTS INTERNATIONAL ORGANIZATION, INC.
Nationwide support group for patients and families
2117 L Street N.W., #353
Washington, DC 20037
Toll-Free: 1-800-TRIO-386
202-293-0980
Web site: www.trioweb.org
Email: triointl@aol.com

UNITED NETWORK FOR ORGAN SHARING (UNOS)
P.O. Box 2484
Richmond, VA 23218
804-782-4800
Toll-Free Patient Information: 1-888-TX INFO1 (894-6361)
Web site: www.unos.org

Note: Multiple Internet sites with information on hemochromatosis exist. Although many have important information, we do not specifically endorse any of these sites although we have used resources from government-based Web sites in the production of this book.

SELECTED CITATION

CHAPTER 1. WHAT IS HEMOCHROMATOSIS?

Bacon, B.R. 2001. Hemochromatosis: Diagnosis and Management. *Gastroenterology*. 120:718–725.

Bacon, B.R. 1989. Joseph H. Sheldon and Hereditary Hemochromatosis: Historical Highlights. *Journal of Laboratory Clinical Medicine*. 113:761–2.

Bothwell, T.H., R.W. Charlton. 1988. "Historical Overview of Hemochromatosis." *Hemochromatosis, Procedings of the First International Conference*. Eds. L. R. Weintrub, C. Q. Edwards, M. Krikker. New York: Annals of the New York Academy of Sciences, 526:1–10.

Byrnes, V., E. Ryan, S. Barrett, P. Kenny, P. Mayne, J. Crowe. 2001. Genetic Hemochromatosis, a Celtic Disease: Is It Now Time for Population Screening? *Genetic Testing*. 5:127–130.

Centers for Disease Control and Prevention. 2000. *HIV/AIDS Surveillance Report*. 12(No.2):5–6.

Cogswell, Mary E., S.M. McDonnell, M.J. Khoury, A. L. Franks, W. Burke, G. Brittenham. 1998. Iron Overload, Public Health, and Genetics: Evaluating the Evidence for Hemochromatosis Screening. *Annals of Internal Medicine*. 129:971–979.

Datz, C., T. Haas, H. Rinner, F. Sandhofer, W. Patsch, B. Paulwever. 1998. Heterozygosity for the C282Y Mutation in the Hemochromatosis Gene Is Associated with Increased Serum Iron, Transferrin Saturation, and Hemoglobin in Young Women: A Protective Role Against Iron Deficiency? *Clinical Chemistry*. 44 (12): 2429–32.

Datz, C., M.R.A. Lalloz, W.Vogel, I. Graziadei, F. Hackl, G.Vautier, D.M. Layton, T. Maier-Dobersberger, P. Ferenci, E. Penner, F. Sandhofer, A. Bomford, B. Paulweber. 1997. Predominance of the HLA-H Cys282Tyr Mutation in Austrian Patients with Genetic Haemochromatosis. *Journal of Hepatology*. 27(5): 773–9.

EASL International Consensus Conference on Haemochromatosis. 2000. *Journal of Hepatology*. 33: 485–504.

Feder, J.N., A. Gnirke, W. Thomas, Z. Tsuchihashi, D.A. Ruddy, A. Basava, F. Dormishian, R. Domingo, Jr., M.C. Ellis, A. Fullan, L.M. Hinton, N.L. Jones, B.E. Kimmel, G.S. Kronmal, P. Lauer, V.K. Lee, D.B. Loeb, F.A. Mapa, E. McClelland,

N.C. Meyer, G.A. Mintier, N. Moeller, T. Moore, E. Morikang, C.E. Prass, L. Quintana, S.M. Starnes, R.C. Schatzman, K.J. Brunke, D.T. Drayna, N.J. Risch, B.R. Bacon & R.K. Wolff. 1996. A Novel MHC Class-I-Like Gene Is Mutated in Patients with Hereditary Haemochromatosis. *Nature Genetics.* 13:399-408.

"Hemochromatosis." March 1999. *National Institute of Diabetes & Digestive & Kidney Diseases.* <www.niddk.nih.gov/health/digest/pubs/hemochom/hemochromatosis.htm.> 30 June 2002.

"Iron Overload Disease Due to Hereditary Hemochromatosis." 23 May 2002. *Centers for Disease Control and Prevention.* <www.cdc.gov/nccdphp/dnpa/hemochromatosis/hereditary.htm> 30 June 2002.

Looker, Anne C., C.L. Johnson. 1998. Prevalence of Elevated Serum Transferrin Saturation in Adults in the United States. *Annals of Internal Medicine.* 129:940-945.

Lucotte, G. 2001. Frequency Analysis and Allele Map in Favor of the Celtic Origin of the C282Y Mutation of Hemochromatosis. *Blood Cells Molecular Disease.* 27:549-556.

McDonnell, Sharon M., P.D. Phatak, V. Felitti, A. Hover, G. McLaren. 1998. Screening for Hemochromatosis in Primary Care Settings. *Annals of Internal Medicine.* 129:962-970.

McDonnell, S.M., B.L. Preston, S.A. Jewell, J.C. Barton, C.Q. Edwards, P.C. Adams, R. Yip. 1999. A Survey of 2,851 Patients with Hemochromatosis: Symptoms and Response to Treatment. *American Journal of Medicine.* 106:619-624.

Parker, Elinor, ed. 1960. *100 More Story Poems.* New York: Thomas Y. Crowell.

Phatak, Pradhyumna D., R.L. Sham, R.F. Raubertas, K. Dunnigan, M.T. O'Leary, C. Braggins, J.D. Cappuccio. 1998. Prevalence of Hereditary Hemochromatosis in 16,031 Primary Care Patients. *Annals of Internal Medicine.* 129:954-961.

Powell, L.W., K. George, S.M. McDonnell, K.V. Kowdley. 1998. Diagnosis of Hemochromatosis. *Annals of Internal Medicine.* 129:925-931.

Powell, L.W., V.N. Subramaniam, T.R. Yapp. 1999. Haemochromatosis In the New Millennium. *Journal of Hepatology.* 32 (suppl. 1): 48-62.

Pozzato, G., F. Zorat, F. Nascimben, M. Gregorutti, C. Comar, S. Baracetti, S. Vatta, E. Bevilacqua, A. Belgrano, S. Crovella, A. Amoroso. 2001. Haemochromatosis Gene Mutations in a Clustered Italian Population: Evidence of High Prevalence in People of Celtic Ancestry. *European Journal of Human Genetics.* 9:445-451.

Sheldon, J.H. 1935. *Haemochromatosis.* London: Oxford University Press.

Sheldon, J.H. 1927. The Iron Content of the Tissues in Haemochromatosis with Special Reference to the Brain. *The Quarterly Journal of Medicine.* 21:123-137.

Simon, M., M. Bourel, R. Fauchet, B. Genetet. 1976. Association of HLA-A3 and HLA-B14 Antigens with Idiopathic Haemochromatosis. *Gut.* 17:332-334.

Tavill, Anthony S. 2001. Diagnosis and Management of Hemochromatosis. *Hepatology.* 33:1321-1328.

CHAPTER 2. WHEN YOU HAVE HEMOCHROMATOSIS

Adams, Paul C., Y. Deugnier, R. Moirand, P. Brissot. 1997. The Relationship between Iron Overload, Clinical Symptoms, and Age in 410 Patients with Genetic Hemochromatosis. *Hepatology.* 25:162-166.

Adams, Paul C., S. Chakrabarti. 1998. Genotypic/Phenotypic Correlations in Genetic Hemochromatosis: Evolution of Diagnostic Criteria. *Gastroenterology.* 114:319-323.

Adams, Paul C., A.E. Kertesz, C.E. McLaren, R. Barr, A. Bamford, S. Chakrabarti. 2000. Population Screening for Hemochromatosis: A Comparison of Unbound Iron Binding Capacity, Transferrin Saturation and C282Y Genotyping in 5,211 Voluntary Blood Donors. *Hepatology.* 31:1160-1164.

Andrews, Nancy C. 1999. Disorders of Iron Metabolism. *New England Journal of Medicine.* 341 (26): 1986-1995.

Bacon, B.R. 2001. Hemochromatosis: Diagnosis and Management. *Gastroenterology.* 120:718-725.

Beaton, Melanie, D. Guyader, Y. Deugnier, R. Moirand, S. Chakrabarti, P. Adams. 2002. Noninvasive Prediction of Cirrhosis in C282Y-Linked Hemochromatosis. *Hepatology.* 36:673-678.

Bonkovsky, Herbert L., D.P. Slaker, E.B. Bills, D.C. Wolf. 1990. Usefulness and Limitations of Laboratory and Hepatic Imaging Studies in Iron-Storage Disease. *Gastroenterology.* 99:1079-1091.

Bravo, Arturo A., S.G. Sheth, S. Chopra. 2001. Liver Biopsy. *New England Journal of Medicine.* 344:495-500.

Deugnier, Yves M., B. Turlin, L.W. Powell, K.W. Summers, R. Moirand, L. Fletcher, O. Loreal, P. Brissot, J.W. Halliday. 1993. Differentiation Between Heterozygotes and Homozygotes in Genetic Hemochromatosis by Means of a Histological Hepatic Iron Index: A Study of 192 Cases. *Hepatology.* 17:30-34.

Dixon, Ruth M., P. Styles, F.N. Al-Refaie, G. J. Kemp, S.M. Donohue, B. Wonke, A.V. Hoffbrand, G.K. Radda, B. Rajagopalan. 1994. Assessment of Hepatic Iron Overload in Thalassemic Patients by Magnetic Resonance Spectroscopy. *Hepatology.* 19:904-910.

Edwards, Corwin Q., L.M. Griffen, D. Goldbar, C. Drummond, M.H. Skolnick, J.P. Kushner. 1988. Prevalence of Hemochromatosis Among 11,065 Presumably Healthy Blood Donors. *New England Journal of Medicine.* 318:1355-1362.

Edwards, Corwin Q., J.P. Kushner. 1993. Screening for Hemochromatosis. *New England Journal of Medicine*. 328:1616-1620.

Guyader, D., Y. Gandon, Y. Deugnier, H. Jouanolle, O. Loreal, M. Simon, M. Bourel, M. Carsin, P. Brissot. 1989. Evaluation of Computed Tomography in the Assessment of Liver Iron Overload. *Gastroenterology*. 97:737-743.

Guyader, D., Y. Gandon, J.Y. Robert, J.F. Heautot, H. Jouanolle, C. Jacquelinet, M. Messner, Y. Deugnier, P. Brissot. 1992. Magnetic Resonance Imaging and Assessment of Liver Iron Content in Genetic Hemochromatosis. *Journal of Hepatology*. 15:304-308.

Kowdley, Kris V., T.D. Trainer, J.R. Saltzman, M. Pedrosa, E.L. Krawitt, T.A. Knox, K. Susskind, D. Pratt, H.L. Bonkovsky, N.D. Grace, M.M. Kaplan. 1997. Utility of Hepatic Iron Index in American Patients with Hereditary Hemochromatosis: A Multicenter Study. *Gastroenterology*. 113:1270-1277.

Looker, Anne C., C.L. Johnson. 1998. Prevalence of Elevated Serum Transferrin Saturation in Adults in the United States. *Annals of Internal Medicine*. 129:940-945.

McLaren, Christine E., G.J. McLachlan, J.W. Halliday, S.I. Webb, B.A. Leggett, E.C. Jazwinska, D.H.G. Crawford, V.R. Gordeuk, G.D. McLaren, L.W. Powell. 1998. Distribution of Transferrin Saturation in an Australian Population: Relevance to the Early Diagnosis of Hemochromatosis. *Gastroenterology*. 114:543-549.

Olynyk, J.K., R. O'Neill, R.S. Britton, B.R. Bacon. 1994. Determination of Hepatic Iron Concentration in Fresh and Paraffin-Embedded Tissue: Diagnostic Implications. *Gastroenterology*. 106:674-677.

Powell, Lawrie W., K.M. Summers, P.G. Board, E. Axelsen, S. Webb, J.W. Halliday. 1990. Expression of Hemochromatosis in Homozygous Subjects: Implications for Early Diagnosis and Prevention. *Gastroenterology*. 98:1625-1632.

Powell, L.W., K. George, S.M. McDonnell, K.V. Kowdley. 1998. Diagnosis of Hemochromatosis. *Annals of Internal Medicine*. 129:925-931.

Rocchi, Emilio, M. Cassanelli, A. Borghi, F. Paolillo, M. Pradelli, G. Casalgrandi, A. Burani, E. Gallo. 1993. Magnetic Resonance Imaging and Different Levels of Iron Overload in Chronic Liver Disease. *Hepatology*. 17:997-1002.

Roudot-Thoraval, Francoise, M. Halphen, D. Larde, M. Galliot, J-C. Rymer, F. Galacteros, D. Dhumeaux. 1983. Evaluation of Liver Iron Content by Computed Tomography: Its Value in the Follow-Up of Treatment in Patients with Idiopathic Hemochromatosis. *Hepatology*. 6:974-979.

Summers, Kim M., J.W. Halliday, L.W. Powell. 1990. Identification of Homozygous Hemochromatosis Subjects by Measurement of Hepatic Iron Index. *Hepatology*. 12:20-25.

Schoniger-Hekele, M., C. Muller, C. Polli, F. Wrba, E. Penner, P. Ferenci. 2002. Liver Pathology in Compound Heterozygous Patients for Hemochromatosis Mutations. *Liver.* 22:295-301.

Tavill, Anthony S. 2001. Diagnosis and Management of Hemochromatosis. *Hepatology.* 33:1321-1328.

CHAPTER 3. GENETIC (DNA) TESTS

Bacon, Bruce R., J.K. Olynyk, E.M. Brunt, R.S. Britton, R.K. Wolff. 1999. HFE Genotype in Patients with Hemochromatosis and Other Liver Diseases. *Annals of Internal Medicine.* 130:953-962.

Bacon, B.R. 2001. Hemochromatosis: Diagnosis and Management. *Gastroenterology.* 120:718-725.

Beutler, E., V.J. Felitti, J.A. Koziol, T. Gelbart. 2002. Penetrance of 845G>A (C282Y) HFE Hereditary Haemochromatosis Mutation in the USA. *Lancet.* 359:211-218.

Bomford, A. 2002. Genetics of Haemochromatosis. *Lancet.* 360:1673-1681.

Burke, Wylie. 2002. Genetic Testing. *New England Journal of Medicine.* 347:1867-1875.

Camaschella, Clara, S. Fargion, M. Sampietro, A. Roetto, S. Bosio, G. Garozzo, C. Arosio, A. Piperno. 1999. Inherited HFE-Unrelated Hemochromatosis in Italian Families. *Hepatology.* 29:1563-1564

El-Serag H.B., J.M. Inadomi, K.V. Kowdley. 2000. Screening for Hereditary Hemochromatosis in Siblings and Children of Affected Patients: A Cost-Effectiveness Analysis. *Annals of Internal Medicine.* 132:261-269.

Gochee, P.A., L.W. Powell, D.J. Cullen, D. Du Sart, E. Rossi, J.K. Olynyk. 2002. A Population-Based Study of the Biochemical and Clinical Expression of the H63D Hemochromatosis Mutation. *Gastroenterology.* 122:646-651.

Guttmacher, Alan E., F. S. Collins. 2002. Genomic Medicine—A Primer. *New England Journal of Medicine.* 347:1512-1520.

"HHS Publishes Final Privacy Rule; Labs Must Comply by April 14, 2003." 14 August 2002. College of American Pathologists. <http://www.cap.org/html/advocacy/statline/HIPAA_Special _Report.html.> 24 Sept. 2002.

Moore, Pete. 2000. *Babel's Shadow, Genetic Technologies in a Fracturing Society.* Oxford: Lion Publishing.

Moirand, Romain, A-M. Jouanolle, P. Brissot, J-Y. Le Gall, V. David, Y. Deugnier. 1999. Phenotypic Expression of HFE Mutations: A French Study of 1,110 Unrelated Iron-Overloaded Patients and Relatives. *Gastroenterology.* 116:372-377.

Olynyk, John K., D.J. Cullen, S. Aquilia, E. Rossi, L. Summerville, L.W. Powell. 1999. A Population-Based Study of the Clinical Expression of the Hemochromatosis Gene. *New England Journal of Medicine*. 341:718-724.

Pietrangelo, Antonello, G. Montosi, A. Totaro, C. Garuti, D. Conte, S. Cassenelli, M. Fraquelli, C. Sardini, F. Vasta, P. Gasparini. 1999. Hereditary Hemochromatosis in Adults without Pathogenic Mutations in the Hemochromatosis Gene. *New England Journal of Medicine*. 341:725-732.

Shaheen, Nicholas J., B.R. Bacon, I.S. Grimm. 1998. Clinical Characteristics of Hereditary Hemochromatosis Patients Who Lack the C282Y Mutation. *Hepatology*. 28:526-529.

Stewart, S.F., C.P. Day. 2001. Liver Disorder and the HFE Locus. *Quarterly Journal of Medicine*. 94:453-456.

Tavill, Anthony S. 1999. Clinical Implications of the Hemochromatosis Gene. *New England Journal of Medicine*. 341:755-757.

Tavill, Anthony S. 2001. Diagnosis and Management of Hemochromatosis. *Hepatology*. 33:1321-1328.

Wallace, Daniel F., J.S. Dooley, A.P. Walker. 1999. A Novel Mutation of HFE Explains the Classical Phenotype of Genetic Hemochromatosis in a C282Y Heterozygote. *Gastroenterology*. 116:1409-1412.

Whiting, P.W., L.M. Fletcher, J.K. Dixon, P. Gochee, L.W. Powell, D.H. Crawford. 2002. Concordance of Iron Indices in Homozygote and Heterozygote Sibling Pairs in Hemochromatosis Families: Implications for Family Screening. *Journal of Hepatology*. 37:309-314.

CHAPTER 4. THE CARRIER

Bathum, L., L. Christiansen, H. Nybo, K.A. Ranberg, D. Gaist, B. Jeune, N.E. Petersen, J. Vaupel, K. Christensen. 2001. Association of Mutations in the Hemochromatosis Gene with Shorter Life Expectancy. *Archives of Internal Medicine*. 161:2441-2444.

Bulaj, Z.J., L.M. Griffen, L.B. Jorde, C. Q. Edwards, J.P. Kushner. 1996. Clinical and Biochemical Abnormalities in People Heterozygous for Hemochromatosis. *New England Journal of Medicine*. 335:1799-1805.

Case Records of the Massachusetts General Hospital. 1997. *New England Journal of Medicine*. 336:939-947.

Crawford, D.H., E.C. Jazwinska, L.M. Cullen, L.W. Powell. 1998. Expression of HLA-Linked Hemochromatosis in Subjects Homozygous or Heterozygous for the C282Y Mutation. *Gastroenterology*. 114:1003-1008.

El-Serag H.B., J.M. Inadomi, K.V. Kowdley. 2000. Screening for Hereditary Hemochromatosis in Siblings and Children of Affected Patients: A Cost-Effectiveness Analysis. *Annals of Internal Medicine.* 132:261–269.

Fuchs, J., M. Podda, L. Packer, R. Kaufmann. 2002. Morbidity Risk in HFE Associated Hereditary Hemochromatosis C282Y Heterozygotes. *Toxicology.* 180:169–181.

Gochee, P.A., L.W. Powell, D.J. Cullen, D. Du Sart, E. Rossi, J.K. Olynyk. 2002. A Population-Based Study of the Biochemical and Clinical Expression of the H63D Hemochromatosis Mutation. *Gastroenterology.* 122:646–651.

Moirand, R., D. Guyader, M.H. Mendler, A.M. Jouanolle, J.Y. Le Gall, V. David, P. Brissot, Y. Deugnier. 2002. HFE Based Re-evaluation of Heterozygous Hemochromatosis. *American Journal of Medical Genetics.* 111:356–361.

Powell, Lawrie W., E.C. Jazwinska. 1996. Hemochromatosis in Heterozygotes. *New England Journal of Medicine.* 335:1837–1839.

Tavill, Anthony S. 2001. Diagnosis and Management of Hemochromatosis. *Hepatology.* 33:1321–1328.

CHAPTER 5. HOW HEMOCHROMATOSIS AFFECTS YOUR BODY

Adams, Paul C., M. Speechley, A.E. Kertesz. 1991. Long-Term Survival Analysis in Hereditary Hemochromatosis. *Gastroenterology.* 101:368–372.

Adams, Paul C., Y. Deugnier, R. Moirand, P. Brissot. 1997. The Relationship between Iron Overload, Clinical Symptoms, and Age in 410 Patients with Genetic Hemochromatosis. *Hepatology.* 25:162–166.

Annichino-Bizzacchi, J.M., S.T. Saad, V R. Arruda, J.A. Ramirez, L.H. Siqueira, L.C. Chiaparini, A.P. Mansur. 2000. C282Y Mutation in the HLA-H Gene Is Not a Risk Factor for Patients with Myocardial Infarction. *Journal of Cardiovascular Risk.* 7:37–40.

Askari, Ali D., W.A. Muir, I.A. Rosner, R.W. Moskowitz, G.D. McLaren, W.E. Braun. 1983. Arthritis of Hemochromatosis. *American Journal of Medicine.* 75:957–965.

Barton, James C., S.M. McDonnell, P.C. Adams, P. Brissot, L.W. Powell, C.Q. Edwards, J.D. Cook, K.V. Kowdley. 1998. Management of Hemochromatosis. *Annals of Internal Medicine.* 129:932–939.

Beaton, Melanie, D. Guyader, Y. Deugnier, R. Moirand, S. Chakrabarti, P. Adams. 2002. Noninvasive Prediction of Cirrhosis in C282Y-Linked Hemochromatosis. *Hepatology.* 36:673–678.

Bergmann T.K., K. Vinding, H. Hey. 2001. Multiple Hepatic Abscesses Due to Yersinia Enterocolitica Infection Secondary to Primary Haemochromatosis. Scandinavian *Journal of Gastroenterology.* 36:891–5.

Beutler, E., V.J. Felitti, J.A. Koziol, T. Gelbart. 2002. Penetrance of 845G>A (C282Y) HFE Hereditary Haemochromatosis Mutation in the USA. *Lancet.* 359:211-218.

Bozzini, C., D. Girelli, E. Tinazzi, O. Olivieri, C. Stranieri, A. Bassi, E. Trabetti, G. Faccini, P.F. Pignatti, R. Corrocher. 2002. Biochemical and Genetic Markers of Iron Status and the Risk of Coronary Artery Disease: An Angiography-Based Study. *Clinical Chemistry.* 48:622-628.

Candell-Riera, J., L. Lu, L. Seres, J.B. Gonzales, J. Batlle, G. Permanyer-Miralda, H. Garcia-del-Castillo, J. Soler-Soler. 1983. Cardiac Hemochromatosis: Beneficial Effects of Iron Removal Therapy. *American Journal of Cardiology.* 52:824-829.

Conte, Dario, A. Piperno, C. Mandelli, S. Fargion, M. Cesana, L. Brunelli, L. Ferrario, P. Velio, M G. Zaramella, C. Tiribelli. 1986. Clinical, Biochemical, and Histological Features of Primary Haemochromatosis: A Report of 67 Cases. *Liver.* 6:310-315.

Conte, Dario, D. Manachino, A. Colli, A. Guala, G. Aimo, M. Andreoletti, M. Corsetti, M. Fraquella. 1998. Prevalence of Genetic Hemochromatosis in a Cohort of Italian Patients with Diabetes Mellitus. *Annals of Internal Medicine.* 128:370-373.

Dabestani, A., J. S. Child, E. Henze, J. K. Perloff, H. Schon, W. G. Figueroa, H. R. Schelbert, S. Thessomboon. 1984. Primary Hemochromatosis: Anatomic and Physiologic Characteristics of the Cardiac Ventricles and Their Response to Phlebotomy. *American Journal of Cardiology.* 54:153-159.

Deugnier, Yves M., O. Loreal, B. Turlin, D. Guyader, H. Jouanolle, R. Moirand, C. Jacquelinet, P. Brissot. 1992. Liver Pathology in Genetic Hemochromatosis: A Review of 135 Homozygous Cases and Their Bioclinical Correlations. *Gastroenterology.* 102:2050-2059.

Diamond, Terrence, D. Stiel, S. Posen. 1989. Osteoporosis in Hemochromatosis: Iron Excess, Gonadal Deficiency, or Other Factors? *Annals of Internal Medicine.* 110:430-436.

Dubois-Laforgue, D., S. Caillat-Zucman, C. Boitard, J. Timsit. 2000. Clinical Characteristics of Type 2 Diabetes in Patients with Mutations of HFE. *Diabetes Metabolism.* 26:65-68.

Fargion, Silvia, C. Mandelli, A. Piperno, B. Cesana, A.L. Fracanzani, M. Fraquelli, P.A. Bianchi, G. Fiorelli, D. Conte. 1992. Survival and Prognostic Factors in 212 Italian Patients with Genetic Hemochromatosis. *Hepatology.* 15:655-659.

Finch, S.C. 1955. Idiopathic Hemochromatosis, An Iron Storage Disease. *Medicine.* 324:381-430.

Gerhard, G.S., K.A. Levin, J. Price-Goldstein, M.M. Wojnar, M.J. Chorney, D. A. Belchis. 2001. Vibrio Vulnificus Septicemia in a Patient with the Hemochromatosis HFE C282Y Mutation. *Archives of Pathology and Laboratory Medicine.* 125:1107-1109.

Hanson, E.H., G. Imperatore, W. Burke. 2001. HFE Gene and Hereditary Hemochromatosis: a HuGE Review, Human Genome Epidemiology. *American Journal of Epidemiology*. 154:193–206.

Jackson, H.A., K. Carter, C. Darke, M.G. Guttridge, D. Ravine, R.D. Hutton, J.A. Napier, M. Worwood. 2001. HFE Mutations, Iron Deficiency and Overload in 10,500 Blood Donors. *British Journal of Haematology*. 114:474–484.

Mahon, N.G., A.S. Coonar, S. Jeffrey, F. Coccolo, J. Akiyu, B. Zal, R. Houlston, G.E. Levin, C. Baboonian, W.J. McKenna. 2000. Haemochromatosis Gene Mutations in Idiopathic Dilated Cardiomyopathy. *Heart*. 84:541–547.

McDonnell, S.M., B.L. Preston, S.A. Jewell, J.C. Barton, C.Q. Edwards, P.C. Adams, R. Yip. 1999. A Survey of 2,851 Patients with Hemochromatosis: Symptoms and Response to Treatment. *American Journal of Medicine*. 106:619–624.

Milman, N., P. Pedersen, T.A. Stieg, K.E. Byg, N. Graudal, K. Fenger. 2001. Clinically Overt Hereditary Hemochromatosis in Denmark 1948–1985: Epidemiology, Factors of Significance for Long-Term Survival, and Causes of Death in 179 Patients. *Annals of Hematology*. 80:737–744.

Moczulski, D.K., W. Grzeszczak, B. Gawlik. 2001. Role of Hemochromatosis C282Y and H63D Mutations in HFE Gene in Development of Type 2 Diabetes and Diabetic Nephropathy. *Diabetes Care*. 24:1187–1191.

Moirand, Romain, P.C. Adams, V. Bicheler, P. Brissot, Y. Deugnier. 1997. Clinical Features of Genetic Hemochromatosis in Women Compared to Men. *Annals of Internal Medicine*. 127:105–110.

Moodie, S.J., L. Ang, J.M. Stenner, C. Finlayson, A. Khotari, G.E. Levin, J.D. Maxwell. 2002. Testing for Haemochromatosis in a Liver Clinic Population: Relationship between Ethnic Origin, HFE Gene Mutations, Liver Histology, and Serum Iron Markers. *European Journal of Gastroenterology and Hepatology*. 14:217–221.

Niederau, Claus, R. Fischer, A. Sonnenberg, W. Stremmel, H.J. Trampisch, G. Strohmeyer. 1985. Survival and Causes of Death in Cirrhotic and Noncirrhotic Patients with Primary Hemochromatosis. *New England Journal of Medicine*. 313:1256–1262.

Niederau, Claus, G. Strohmeyer, W. Stremmel. 1994. Epidemiology, Clinical Spectrum, and Prognosis of Hemochromatosis. *Advances in Experimental Medicine and Biology*. 356:293–302.

Niederau, Claus, R. Fischer, A. Purschel, W. Stremmel, D. Haussinger, G. Strohmeyer. 1996. Long-Term Survival in Patients with Hereditary Hemochromatosis. *Gastroenterology*. 110:1107–1119.

Njajou, O.T., M. Hollander, P.J. Koudstaal, A. Hofman, J.C. Witteman, M.M. Breteler, C. M. van Duijn. 2002. Mutations in the Hemochromatosis Gene (HFE) and Stroke. *Stroke*. 33:2363–2366.

Olson L.J., W.D. Edwards, D.R. Holmes, Jr, F.A. Miller, Jr, L.A. Nordstrom, W.P. Baldus. 1989. Endomyocardial Biopsy in Hemochromatosis: Clinicopathologic Correlates in Six Cases. *Journal of the American College of Cardiology.* 13:116-120.

Olson L.J., W.P. Baldus, A.J. Tajik. 1987. Echocardiographic Features of Idiopathic Hemochromatosis. *American Journal of Cardiology.* 60:885-9.

Rasmussen, M.L., A.R. Folsom, D.J. Catellier, M.Y. Tsai, U. Garg, J.H. Eckfeldt. 2001. A Prospective Study of Coronary Heart Disease and the Hemochromatosis Gene (HFE) C282Y Mutation: The Atherosclerosis Risk in Communities (ARIC) Study. *Atherosclerosis.* 154:739-746.

Roest, M., Y.T. van der Schouw, B. de Valk, J.J. Marx, M J. Tempelman, P.G. de Groot, J J. Sixma, J.D. Banga. 1999. Heterozygosity for a Hereditary Hemochromatosis Gene Is Associated with Cardiovascular Death in Women. *Circulation.* 100:1268-1273.

Salonen, Jukka T., T-P. Tuomainen, K. Kontula. 2000. Role of C282Y Mutation in Haemochromatosis Gene in Development of Type 2 Diabetes in Healthy Men: Prospective Cohort Study. *British Medical Journal.* 320:1706-1707.

Sampietro, M., G. Fiorelli, S. Fargion. 1999. Iron Overload in Porphyria Cutanea Tarda. *Haematologica.* 84:248-253.

Sampson, M.J., T. Williams, P.J. Heyburn, R.H. Greenwood, R.C. Temple, J.Z. Wimperis, B.A. Jennings, G.A. Willis. 2000. Prevalence of HFE (Hemochromatosis Gene) Mutations in Unselected Male Patients with Type 2 Diabetes. *Journal of Laboratory and Clinical Medicine.* 135:170-173.

Smith, Lloyd H. 1990. Overview of Hemochromatosis. *Western Journal of Medicine.* 153:296-308.

Strohmeyer, G., C. Niederau, W. Stremmel. 1988. Survival and Cause of Death in Hemochromatosis: Observations in 163 Patients. *Annals of the New York Academy of Sciences.* 526:245-257.

Timms, A.E., R. Sathananthan, L. Bradbury, N.A. Athanasou, M..A. Brown. 2002. Genetic Testing for Haemochromatosis in Patients with Chondrocalcinosis. *Annals of Rheumatologic Diseases.* 61:745-747.

Tuomainen, T.P., K. Kontula, K. Nyyssonen, T.A. Lakka, T. Helio, J.T. Salonen. 1999. Increased Risk of Acute Myocardial Infarction in Carriers of the Hemochromatosis Gene Cys282Tyr Mutation: A Prospective Cohort Study in Men in Eastern Finland. *Circulation.* 100:1260-1263.

Van Lerberghe, S., M.P. Hermans, K. Dahan, M. Bursschaert. 2002. Clinical Expression and Insulin Sensitivity in Type 2 Diabetic Patients with Heterozygous Mutations for Haemochromatosis. *Diabetes Metabolism.* 28:33-38.

Waalen, J., V. Felitti, T. Gelbart, N.J. Ho, E. Beutler. 2002. Prevalence of Coronary

Heart Disease Associated with HFE Mutations in Adults Attending a Health Appraisal Center. *American Journal of Medicine.* 113:472–479.

Willis, G., J.Z. Wimperis, R. Lonsdale, I.W. Fellows, M.A. Watson, L.M. Skipper, B.A. Jennings. 2000. Incidence of Liver Disease in People with HFE Mutations. *Gut.* 46:401–404.

Yang, Quanhe, S.M. McDonnell, M.J. Khoury, J. Cono, R.G. Parrish. 1998. Hemochromatosis-Associated Mortality in the United States from 1979 to 1992: An Analysis of Multiple-Cause Mortality Data. *Annals of Internal Medicine.* 129:946–953.

CHAPTER 6. TAKING CARE OF YOURSELF NUTRITIONALLY

Barton, James C., S.M. McDonnell, P.C. Adams, P. Brissot, L.W. Powell, C.Q. Edwards, J.D. Cook, K.V. Kowdley. 1998. Management of Hemochromatosis. *Annals of Internal Medicine.* 129:932–939.

Garrison, Cheryl. 2001. *Cooking with Less Iron.* Nashville: Cumberland House Publishing.

Marquis, Christopher. 2000. "90% of U.S. Diets Lacking, Feds Say." *Denver Post.* 28 May, 24A.

Munoz, S.J. 1991. Nutritional Therapies in Liver Disease. *Seminars in Liver Disease.* 11:278–291.

Nompleggi, D.J., H.L. Bonkovsky. 1994. Nutritional Supplementation in Chronic Liver Disease: An Analytical Review. *Hepatology.* 19:518–533.

"On the Home Front." Nov.-Dec. 1997, rev. June 2002. U.S. Food and Drug Administration. 12 Dec. 2002. <http://www.cfsan.fda.gov/~dms/fdsafe4.html.>

"Q and A's on Dietary Guidelines for Americans, 2000." 3 June 2000. *Center for Nutrition Policy and Promotion.* 1 Sept. 2000. http://www.usda.gov/cnpp/Pubs/DG2000/ Qa5-2.pdf.>

U.S. Department of Agriculture, U.S. Department of Health and Human Services. 1995. *Dietary Guidelines for Americans.* Fourth Edition. Washington.

U.S. Food and Drug Administration. May 1993. *Important Health Information for People with Immune Disorders.* DHHS Publication No. (FDA) 93-2267. Washington.

U.S. Food and Drug Administration. Feb. 8, 1993. *Advice on Consumption of Raw Molluscan Shellfish.* FDA Fact Sheet. Washington.

CHAPTER 7. TAKING CARE OF YOURSELF EMOTIONALLY

Anderson, Greg. 1993. *50 Essential Things to Do When the Doctor Says It's Cancer.* New York: Plume/Penguin.

Benson, Herbert with Marg Stark. 1996. *Timeless Healing, the Power and Biology of Belief.* New York: Scribner.

Benson, Herbert with Miriam Z. Klipper. 1975. *The Relaxation Response.* New York: Avon.

LeShan, Lawrence. 1994. *Cancer As a Turning Point.* New York. Plume/Penguin.

McDonnell, S.M., B.L. Preston, S.A. Jewell, J.C. Barton, C.Q. Edwards, P.C. Adams, R.Yip. 1999. A Survey of 2,851 Patients with Hemochromatosis: Symptoms and Response to Treatment. *American Journal of Medicine.* 106:619-624.

Moore, Pete. 2000. *Babel's Shadow, Genetic Technologies in a Fracturing Society.* Oxford: Lion Publishing.

Moyers, Bill. 1993. *Healing and the Mind.* New York: Doubleday.

Spiegel, David, M.D. 1993. *Living Beyond Limits.* New York: Random House.

Tibben, A.M. Vegter-v.d.Vlis, M.F. Niermeijer, J.J.P. v.d. Kamp, R.A.C. Roos, H.G.M. Rooijmans, P.G. Frets, F. Verhage. 1990. Testing for Huntington's Disease with Support for All Parties. *Lancet.* 335: 553.

Topf, Linda Noble with Hal Z. Bennett. 1995. *You Are Not Your Illness.* New York: Fireside.

CHAPTER 8. FINANCIAL IMPACT OF HEMOCHROMATOSIS

Beam, Jr., Burton T. and Kenn B. Tacchino. Jan. 1997. The Health Insurance Portability and Accountability Act of 1996. *Journal of the American Society of CLU & ChFC.* 14+.

"EEOC Settles ADA Suit Against BNSF for Genetic Bias." 18 April 2001. *U.S. Equal Employment Opportunity Commission.* <http://www.eeoc.gov/press/4-18-01.html.> 9 Sept. 2002.

Gianaro, Catherine. DNA on Trial. *University of Georgia Research Magazine.* Summer 2002, 16-19.

Hall, Mark A., Stephen S. Rich. 2000. Laws Restricting Insurers' Use of Genetic Information: Impact on Genetic Discrimination. *American Journal of Human Genetics.* 66:293-307.

Hall, Mark A. 2000. Patients' Fear of Genetic Discrimination by Health Insurers: The Impact of Legal Protections. *Genetics in Medicine.* 2(4): 214-221.

McDonnell, S.M., A.J. Grindon, B.L. Preston, J.C. Barton, C.Q. Edwards, P.D. Adams. A 1999. A Survey of Phlebotomy among Persons with Hemochromatosis. *Transfusion.* 39:651-656.

McDonnell, S.M., B.L. Preston, S.A. Jewell, J.C. Barton, C.Q. Edwards, P.C. Adams, R.Yip. 1999. A Survey of 2,851 Patients with Hemochromatosis: Symptoms and Response to Treatment. *American Journal of Medicine.* 106:619–624.

Moore, Pete. 2000. *Babel's Shadow, Genetic Technologies in a Fracturing Society.* Oxford: Lion Publishing.

Social Security Administration. Feb. 2002. *Social Security Disability Benefits.* SSA Publication No. 05-10029.

Social Security Administration. March 2001. *Social Security Supplemental Security Income.* SSA Publication No. 05-11000.

Social Security Administration. Sept. 2000. *Understanding Supplemental Income.* SSA Publication No. 17-008.

U.S. Department of Health and Human Services. Centers for Medicare & Medicaid Services. Sept. 2002. *Medicare & You* 2003. Publication No. CMS 10050.

U.S. Department of Health and Human Services. Centers for Medicare & Medicaid Services. Feb. 2002. *2002 Guide to Health Insurance for People with Medicare: Choosing a Medigap Policy.* Publication No. CMS-02110.

U.S. Department of Labor Employment Standards Administration, Wage and Hour Division. Dec. 1996. Publication 1421. *Compliance Guide to the Family and Medical Leave Act.* Washington: U.S. Government Printing Office.

U.S. Department of Labor Employment Standards Administration, Wage and Hour Division. April 1995. WH Publication 1419. Federal Regulations Part 825. *The Family and Medical Leave Act of 1993.* Washington: U.S. Government Printing Office.

U.S. Department of Labor Employment Standards Administration, Wage and Hour Division. June 1993. WH Publication 1420. *Your Rights Under the Family and Medical Leave Act of 1993.* Washington: U.S. Government Printing Office.

U.S. Department of Labor Program. 1993. *The Family and Medical Leave Act of 1993.* Highlights Fact Sheet No. ESA 93-2. Washington: U.S. Government Printing Office.

U.S. Equal Employment Opportunity Commission, U.S. Department of Justice, Civil Rights Division. 1992. *The Americans with Disabilities Act, Questions and Answers.* Washington.

U.S. Equal Employment Opportunity Commission. 1991. *The Americans With Disabilities Act.* Washington.

United Network for Organ Sharing (UNOS). 1997. *What Every Patient Needs to Know.*

CHAPTER 9. TREATMENT FOR HEMOCHROMATOSIS

Bacon, B.R. 2001. Hemochromatosis: Diagnosis and Management. *Gastroenterology*. 120:718-725.

Barton, James C., S.M. McDonnell, P.C. Adams, P. Brissot, L.W. Powell, C.Q. Edwards, J.D. Cook, K.V. Kowdley. 1998. Management of Hemochromatosis. *Annals of Internal Medicine*. 129:932-939.

"Facts About Blood and Blood Banking." January 2002. American Association of Blood Banks. <http://www.aabb.org/All_About_Blood/FAQx/aabb_faqs.htm.> 11 October 2002.

Guthrie, Douglas, M.D., F.R.C.S.Ed., F.R.S.E. 1946. *A History of Medicine*. Philadelphia: J. B. Lippincott Company.

Haggard, Howard W. 1934. *The Doctor in History*. New Haven: Yale University Press.

King, Lester S., M.D. 1982. *Medical Thinking, A Historical Preface*. Princeton: Princeton University Press.

Lasagna, Louis, M.D. 1962. *The Doctors' Dilemmas*. New York: Harper & Brothers.

McDonnell, S.M., A.J. Grindon, B.L. Preston, J.C. Barton, C.Q. Edwards, P.C. Adams. 1999. A Survey of Phlebotomy among Persons with Hemochromatosis. *Transfusion*. 39:651-656.

Tavill, Anthony S. 2001. Diagnosis and Management of Hemochromatosis. *Hepatology*. 33:1321-1328.

"Variances for Blood Collection from Individuals with Hereditary Hemochromatosis." August 2001. Food and Drug Administration. <www.fda.gov/cber/gdlns/hemchrom.htm.> 9 September 2002.

CHAPTER 10. CANCER AND OTHER LIVER COMPLICATIONS

Achkar, J-P., V. Araya, R.L. Baron, J.W. Marsh, I. Dvorchik, J. Rakela. 1998. Undetected Hepatocellular Carcinoma: Clinical Features and Outcome After Liver Transplantation. *Liver Transplantation and Surgery*. Vol. 4, No. 6 (Nov.):477-482.

Bacon, Bruce R., J.K. Olynyk, E.M. Brunt, R.S. Britton, R.K. Wolff. 1999. HFE Genotype in Patients with Hemochromatosis and Other Liver Diseases. *Annals of Internal Medicine*. 130:953-962.

Bruix, J. 1997. Treatment of Hepatocellular Carcinoma. *Hepatology*. 25:259-261.

Chitturi, Shivakumar, M. Weltman, G.C. Farrell, D. MacDonald, C. Liddle, D. Samarasinghe, R. Lin, S. Abeygunasekera, J. George. 2002. HFE Mutations, Hepatic Iron, and Fibrosis: Ethnic-Specific Association of NASH with C282Y but Not with Fibrotic Severity. *Hepatology*. 36:142-149.

Collier, J., M. Sherman. 1998. Screening for Hepatocellular Carcinoma. *Hepatology*. 27:273-278.

Deugnier, Yves M., D. Guyader, L. Crantock, J-M. Lopez, B. Turlin, J. Yaouanq, H. Jouanolle, J-P. Campion, B. Launois, J. W. Halliday, L. W. Powell, P. Brissot. 1993. Primary Liver Cancer in Genetic Hemochromatosis: A Clinical, Pathological, and Pathogenetic Study of 54 Cases. *Gastroenterology*. 104:228-234.

Di Bisceglie, Adrian M., R.L. Carithers, Jr., G.J. Gores. 1998. Hepatocellular Carcinoma. *Hepatology*. 28:1161-1165.

Dorak, M.T., A.K. Burnett, M. Worwood. 2002. Hemochromatosis Gene in Leukemia and Lymphoma. *Leukemia and Lymphoma*. 43:467-477.

Everson, G.T. 2000. Increasing Incidence and Pretransplantation Screening of Hepatocellular Carcinoma. *Liver Transplantation.* Vol. 6, No. 6, Suppl. 2 (Nov.):S2-S10.

Fracanzani, Anna L., D. Conte, M. Fraquelli, E. Taioli, M. Mattioli, A. Losco, S. Fargion. 2001. Increased Cancer Risk in a Cohort of 230 Patients with Hereditary Hemochromatosis in Comparison to Matched Control Patients with Non–Iron-Related Chronic Liver Disease. *Hepatology*. 33:647-651.

George, D. K., S. Goldwurm, G.A. MacDonald, L.L. Cowley, N I. Walker, P.J. Ward, E.C. Jazwinska, L.W. Powell. 1998. Increased Hepatic Iron Concentration in Nonalcoholic Steatohepatitis Is Associated with Increased Fibrosis. *Gastroenterology*. 114:311-318.

Hohler, T., S. Leininger, H.H. Kohler, P. Schirmacher, P.R. Galle. 2000. Heterozygosity for the Hemochromatosis Gene in Liver Diseases—Prevalence and Effects on Liver Histology. *Liver.* 20:482-486.

Lauret, E., M. Rodriguez, S. Gonzalez, A. Linares, A. Lopez-Vazquez, J. Martinez-Borra, C. Lopez-Larrea. 2002. HFE Gene Mutations in Alcoholic- and Virus-Related Cirrhotic Patients with Hepatocellular Carcinoma. *American Journal of Gastroenterology*. 97:1016-1021.

Llovet, J.M., M. Sala, J. Bruix. 2000. Nonsurgical Treatment of Hepatocellular Carcinoma. *Hepatology*. 6 (Suppl 2):S11-S15.

MacDonald, G.A., J. Tarish, V.J. Whitehall, S.J. McCann, G.D. Mellick, R.L. Buttenshaw, A.G. Johnson, J. Young, B.A. Leggett. 1999. No Evidence of Increased Risk of Colorectal Cancer in Individuals Heterozygous for the Cys282Tyr Haemochromatosis Mutation. *Journal of Gastroenterology and Hepatology*. 14:1188-1191.

Mallory, Mark A., K.V. Kowdley. 2001. Hereditary Hemochromatosis and Cancer Risk: More Fuel to the Fire? *Gastroenterology*. 121:1253-1254.

Mazzaferro, V., E. Regalia, R. Doci, S. Andreola, A. Pulvirenti, F. Bozzetti, F. Montalto, M. Ammatuna, A. Morabito, L. Gennari. 1996. Liver Transplantation for the Treatment of Small Hepatocellular Carcinomas in Patients With Cirrhosis. *New*

England Journal of Medicine. 334:693-699.

McMahon, B.J., T. London. 1991. Workshop on Screening for Hepatocellular Carcinoma. *Journal of the National Cancer Institute.* Vol. 83, No. 13 (July 3):916-919.

Penn, I. 1991. Hepatic Transplantation for Primary and Metastatic Cancers of the Liver. *Surgery.* 110:726-734.

Shaheen, N.J., L.M. Silverman, T. Keku, L.B. Lawrence, E.M. Rohlfs, C.F. Martin, J. Galanko, R.S. Sandler. 2003. Association between Hemochromatosis (HFE) Gene Mutation Carrier Status and the Risk of Colon Cancer. *Journal of the National Cancer Institute.* 95:154-159.

Smith, B C., J. Gorve, M.A. Guzail, C.P. Day, A.K. Daly, A D. Burt, M.F. Bassendine. 1998. Heterozygosity for Hereditary Hemochromatosis Is Associated with More Fibrosis in Chronic Hepatitis C. *Hepatology.* 27:1695-1699.

Takayama, T., M. Makuuchi, S. Hirohashi, M. Sakamoto, J. Yamamoto, K. Shimada, T. Kosuge, S. Okada, K. Takayasu, S. Yamasaki. 1998. Early Hepatocellular Carcinoma as an Entity with a High Rate of Surgical Cure. *Hepatology.* 28:1241-1246.

Thornburn, D., G. Curry, R. Spooner, E. Spence, K. Oien, D. Halls, R. Fox, E.A. McCruden, R.N. MacSween, P.R. Mills. 2002. The Role of Iron and Haemochromatosis Gene Mutations in the Progression of Liver Disease in Chronic Hepatitis C. *Gut.* 50:248-252.

Wall, W.J., P.J. Marotta. 2000. Surgery and Transplantation for Hepatocellular Cancer. *Hepatology.* 6 (Suppl 2):S16-S22.

Williams, R., P. Rizzi. 1996. Treating Small Hepatocellular Carcinomas. *New England Journal of Medicine.* Vol. 334, No. 11:728-729.

Wong, L.L., W.M. Limm, R. Severino, L.M. Wong. 2000. Improved Survival with Screening for Hepatocellular Carcinoma. *Liver Transplantation.* Vol. 6, No. 3 (May):320-325.

World Health Organization. *Prevention of Liver Cancer.* Technical Report Series 691. Geneva: WHO, 1983.

Yang, Quanhe, S.M. McDonnell, M.J. Khoury, J. Cono, R.G. Parrish. 1998. Hemochromatosis-Associated Mortality in the United States from 1979 to 1992: An Analysis of Multiple-Cause Mortality Data. *Annals of Internal Medicine.* 129:946-953.

Yuen, M-F, C-C. Cheng, I.J. Lauder, S-K. Lam, C. G-C. Ooi, C-L. Lai. 2000. Early Detection of Hepatocellular Carcinoma Increases the Chance of Treatment: Hong Kong Experience. *Hepatology.* 31:330-335.

CHAPTER 11. LIVER TRANSPLANTS FOR HEMOCHROMATOSIS

Alanen, Kenneth W., S. Chakrabarti, J.J. Rawlins, W. Howson, G. Jeffrey, P.C. Adams. 1999. Prevalence of the C282Y Mutation of the Hemochromatosis Gene in Liver Transplant Recipients and Donors. *Hepatology*. 30:665–669.

Brandhagen, David J., W. Alvarez, T.M. Therneau, K.E. Kruckeberg, S.N. Thibodeau, J. Ludwig, M.K. Porayko. 2000. Iron Overload in Cirrhosis—HFE Genotypes and Outcome After Liver Transplantation. *Hepatology* 31:456-460.

Cotler, Scott J., M.P. Bronner, R.D. Press, T.H. Carlson, J.D. Perkins, M.J. Emond, K.V. Kowdley. 1998. End-Stage Liver Disease without Hemochromatosis Associated with Elevated Hepatic Iron Index. *Journal of Hepatology*. 29:257-262.

Everson, G.T., I. Kam. 2001. Immediate Postoperative Care. In *Transplantation of the Liver*. Editors Maddrey, W.C., E.R. Schiff, M.F. Sorrell. Philadelphia: Lippincott Williams & Wilkins. pp. 131–162.

Everson, Gregory T., J. Trotter. 2002. Liver Transplantation. In *Diseases of the Liver*, Editors Maddrey, W.C., E.R. Schiff, M.F. Sorrell. Philadelphia: Lippincott Williams & Wilkins.

Farrell, Frank J., M. Nguyen, S. Woodley, J C. Imperial, R. Garcia-Kennedy, K. Man, C.O. Esquivel, E.B. Keeffe. 1994. Outcome of Liver Transplantation in Patients with Hemochromatosis. *Hepatology*. 20:404-410.

Fiel, M. Isabel, T.D. Schiano, H.C. Bodenheimer, Jr., S. N. Thung, T.W. King, C.R. Varma, C.M. Miller, E.M. Brunt, S. Starnes, C. Prass, R.K. Wolff, B.R. Bacon. 1999. Hereditary Hemochromatosis in Liver Transplantation. *Liver Transplantation*. 5:50-56.

Halme, L., T. Helio, J. Makinen, K. Hockerstedt, M. Farkkila, K. Piippo, T. Krusius, K. Kontula. 2001. HFE Haemochromatosis Gene Mutations in Liver Transplant Patients. *Scandinavian Journal of Gastroenterology*. 36:881-885.

Ludwig, J., E. Hashimoto, M.K. Porayko, T.P. Moyer, W.P. Baldus. 1997. Hemosiderosis in Cirrhosis: A Study of 447 Native Livers. *Gastroenterology*. 112:882-888.

Olivieri, Nancy F., P.P. Liu, G.D. Sher, P.A. Daly, P. D. Greig, P.J. McCusker, A.F. Collins, W.H. Francombe, D.M. Templeton, J. Butany. 1994. Brief Report: Combined Liver and Heart Transplantation for End-Stage Iron-Induced Organ Failure in an Adult with Homozygous beta-Thalassemia. *New England Journal of Medicine*. 330:1125-1127.

Poulos, J.E., B.R. Bacon. 1996. Liver Transplantation for Hereditary Hemochromatosis. *Digestive Diseases and Sciences*. 14:316-322.

Tung, Bruce Y., F.J. Farrell, T.M. McCashland, R.G. Gish, B.R. Bacon, E.B. Keeffe, K.V. Kowdley. 1999. Long-Term Follow-Up After Liver Transplantation in Patients with Hepatic Iron Overload. *Liver Transplantation*. 5:369-374.

UNOS OPTN and Scientific Registry Data. From the Organ Procurement and Transplantation Network and the US Scientific Registry of Transplant Recipients, www.unos.org, January 2003.

CHAPTER 12. RESEARCH TRENDS

Adams, Paul C. 1999. Population Screening for Hemochromatosis. *Hepatology*. 29:1324–1327.

Adams, Paul C., A.E. Kertesz, C.E. McLaren, R. Barr, A. Bamford, S. Chakrabarti. 2000. Population Screening for Hemochromatosis: A Comparison of Unbound Iron Binding Capacity, Transferrin Saturation and C282Y Genotyping in 5,211 Voluntary Blood Donors. *Hepatology*. 31:1160–1164.

Brittenham, Gary M., A.L. Franks, F.R. Rickles. 1998. Research Priorities in Hereditary Hemochromatosis. *Annals of Internal Medicine*. 129:993–996.

Cogswell, Mary E., S.M. McDonnell, M.J. Khoury, A.L. Franks, W. Burke, G. Brittenham. 1998. Iron Overload, Public Health, and Genetics: Evaluating the Evidence for Hemochromatosis Screening. *Annals of Internal Medicine*. 129:971–979.

Crawford, Darrell H G., P. Hickman. 2000. Screening for Hemochromatosis. *Hepatology*. 31:1192–1193

Cuthbert, Jennifer A. 1997. Iron, HFE, and Hemochromatosis Update. *Journal of Investigative Medicine*. 45:518–529.

El-Serag H. B., J.M. Inadomi, K.V. Kowdley. 2000. Screening for Hereditary Hemochromatosis in Siblings and Children of Affected Patients: A Cost-Effectiveness Analysis. *Annals of Internal Medicine*. 132:261–269.

Hediger, Matthias A., A. Rolfs, T. Goswami. 2002. Iron Transport and Hemochromatosis. *Journal of Investigative Medicine*. 50:239S–246S.

Khoury, Muin J., L.L. McCabe, E R.B. McCabe. 2003. Population Screening in the Age of Genomic Medicine. *New England Journal of Medicine*. 348:50–58.

McDonnell, Sharon M., P.D. Phatak, V. Felitti, A. Hover, G. McLaren. 1998. Screening for Hemochromatosis in Primary Care Settings. *Annals of Internal Medicine*. 129:962–970.

Philpott, Caroline C. 2002. Molecular Aspects of Iron Absorption: Insights into the Role of HFE in Hemochromatosis. *Hepatology*. 35:993–1001.

Tavill, Anthony S. 2001. Diagnosis and Management of Hemochromatosis. *Hepatology*. 33:1321–1328.

Wetterhall, Scott F., M.E. Cogswell, K.V. Kowdley. 1998. Public Health Surveillance for Hereditary Hemochromatosis. *Annals of Internal Medicine*. 129:980–986.

INDEX

A

Abdominal discomfort, 6, 68
Abnormal liver tests, 25, 68, 69
Absorption of iron, 9, 80–81
Aceruloplasminemia, 12
Advanced viral hepatitis, 12
African iron overload, 11
Alanine aminotransferase, 25
Albumin, 26–27
Alcoholic cirrhosis, 12
Alcoholic liver disease, 12
Alcohol injection, 169
Alcohol usage, 7, 63–64, 83
Aldactone, 97
Alkaline phosphatase, 25
Alpha-fetoprotein, 27, 164
ALT (SGPT), 25, 26
American Diabetes Association, 203
American Heart Association National
    Center, 203
American Hemochromatosis Society,
    117, 202
American Liver Foundation, 203
Americans with Disabilities Act of
    1990, 140–141
Amiloride, 97
Anemia, 11
Animal and cell culture models,
    200–201
Apathy, 6, 68
Apple juice, drinking of, 82

Arthritis, 6, 76
Arthritis Foundation, 203
Ascites, 70, 173
Aspartate aminotransferase, 25
AST (SGOT), 25, 26
Azathioprine, 183

B

Balanced diet, eating a, 81, 88–90
Bile, role of, 92
Biliary infection, 77
Bilirubin, 26
Biopsy results, interpretation of, 23–24
Blood banks and patients with
    hemochromatosis, 153–155
Blood removal. See Phlebotomy
Body weight, ideal, 87–88
Bone thinning, 76
"Bronze diabetes," 8
Bronze tone to skin, 6. See also Skin
    pigmentation
Bruising, 6, 69

C

Calcium deficiency, 96
Canadian Hemochromatosis Society,
    202
CAP. See College of American Pathol-

ogists

Carbohydrate metabolism, 91

Cardiac catheterization, 28

Cardiac dysfunction, 72–73

Cardiac studies, 28

Cardiomyopathy and hemochromatosis, 61–62

Carriers

  alcohol use, and, 63–64

  chromosomal implications, 33

  C282Y, issues relevant to, 190–191

  defined, 49, 50

  determination of status, 10–11, 64

  genetic interpretations, 50–53, 54–56, 58–60

  hereditary implications, 60

  HFE gene, 35

  iron supplementation, and, 63–64

  risk factors for iron overload and organ damage, 61–63

  statistical frequency, 4, 50, 51

  vitamin C supplementation and, 63–64

Cast-iron skillets, use of, 83

CBC. See Complete blood count

Cellcept, 183

Celtic populations, occurrence in, 2–3, 4

Centers for Disease Control and Prevention (CDC), 204

Centers for excellence, 192

Chelation costs, 125

Chemoembolization, 168

Chemotherapy, 169

Chromosomes, 9, 10, 17, 32–33

Chronic hepatitis C, 12, 69

Cirrhosis, 28, 68, 69, 160, 161

Cirrhotic patients, 94–97

  caloric requirements, 94–95

  mineral supplementation, 96

  protein restriction, 95–96

  salt and fluid restriction, 96–97

  vitamin supplementation, 96

Clotting factors, 27

Codon, 33

College of American Pathologists, 45

Complete blood count, 27–28

Compound heterozygote, 35–36

Computed tomography (CT), 18, 19, 165

Concentration, lack of, 6

Congenital atransferrinemia, 12

Coordinated care, importance of, 113–114

Cost-effectivness of screening, 197–198

Costs of treatment. See Financial considerations

Counseling, genetic, 38–39

Creative spirit, finding your, 120–121

Cryosurgery, 169

Cyclosporine, 183, 186

C282Y mutations, 4, 9, 17, 18, 34, 35, 48

D

Dcytb, 200

Defined, 1, 10–11

Depression, 103, 110–111

Detection, importance of early, 2, 12

Development of hemochromatosis, 2

Diabetes mellitus, 6, 29, 68, 73, 75

Diagnostic testing. See Testing for hemochromatosis

Diarrheal disease, 77

Dilated capillaries, 69

Disability, applying for, 133–137

Discovery of hemochromatosis, 8

Discrimination, genetic, 105–106, 137–142

Diuretics, use of, 70

DMT1, 200

DNA, role of, 33

Donor livers, 178–179

E

Echocardiogram, 28
E coli, 77
Edema, 26, 70
Emotional considerations
    boundaries, creation of, 112–113
    coordinated care, importance of,
        113–114
    creative spirit, finding your, 120–121
    depression, 103, 110–111
    diagnosis stage, 101–106
    discrimination, genetic, 105–106
    exercise and nutrition, importance
        of, 118
    family systems, role of, 105, 111–113
    frustration, feelings of, 104
    genetic counseling, 114–115
    genetic information overload,
        104–105
    healing *versus* curing, 109–110
    impact phase, 106–108
    implications, 99–101
    isolation, sense of, 104
    life changes, reported, 108
    purpose in our lives, having a sense,
        118–120
    reorganization phase, 109
    research trends and resources, use of,
        115–116
    spiritual self, finding your, 120–121
    support groups, use of, 116–118
    theological challenges, 121
    uncertainty, sense of, 105
Encephalopathy, 71–72, 173
Endocrine system dysfunction, 29,
    73–75
Endomyocardial biopsy, 28
Energy, lack of, 5, 6, 68
Enlarged liver, discovery of, 68
Exercise and nutrition, importance of,
    118

F

Families HHelping Families, 117
Family systems, role of, 105, 111–113
Fatigue, 5, 6, 68
Fat metabolism, 92
Fatty liver, 12, 69
Fecal color, 26
Feder, J.N., 9
Fee-for-service policies, 128–129
Ferrireductase (Dcytb), 200
Ferritin, 16–17, 18
Ferroportin 1 (FP1), 200
Financial considerations
    chelation costs, 125
    disability, applying for, 133–137
    discrimination in insurance and
        employment, genetic,
        137–142
    government health insurance,
        131–132
    Medicaid, 132
    Medicare, 132
    ongoing medical care costs, 125–127
    phlebotomy costs, 124–125
    private health insurance, 127–131
    short-term disability leave,
        133—134
    social security disability insurance,
        135–136
    supplemental security income,
        136–137
    treatment costs, 124–127
    Veterans Administration, 132
Fluid accumulation, 6, 69
Fluids, drinking of, 81
Food labels, importance of, 82
FP1, 200
Fruits and vegetables, importance of
    eating, 82
Fungi, 77
Furosemide, 97

G

Gamma-glutamyl transferase, 25
Genes, role of, 33, 34
Genetic Alliance, 203
Genetic counseling, 38–39, 114–115
Genetic discrimination, 105–106,
    137–142
Genetic information overload,
    104–105
Genetic interpretations, 50–53, 54–56,
    58–60
Genetic mutation, definition of, 10
Genetic testing
    accuracy, 45
    confidentiality of results, 46
    cost of, 44
    defined, 17–18
    extent of testing, determination of,
        43–44
    HFE gene, 30
    HH gene, 30
    HH testing, 44
    implications of, 46
    interpretation of results, 39–43, 45
    recommendations, 53–54, 56–58
    role of, 36–37
    who should be tested?, 37–38
Genotype and phenotype, relationship
    between, 195
GGT, 25, 26
Gnirke, A., 9
Government health insurance, 131–132
Guided imagery, use of, 120

H

HCTZ, 97
H63D mutation, 9, 17, 35, 48
Health Insurance Portability and
    Accountability Act of 1996,
138–139
Heart, complications of the, 72–73
Heart enlargement, 68
Heart rhythm irregularity, 6
Hemochromatosis Foundation, Inc.,
    202
Hemosiderin storage, 15
Hepatic abscess, 77
Hepatic iron index, 68
Hepatic resection, 166
Hepatitis C, chronic, 12, 69
Hepatitis vaccinations, 82
Hepatoma. See Liver cancer
Hepcidin, 200
Hereditary implications, 60
Heterozygote, 35
HFE gene, 1, 2, 4, 9, 10, 17–18, 30, 34,
    35–36, 200
HH gene, 30, 44
High-frequency radio waves, treatment
    with, 168
HII. See Hepatic iron index
Histologic stages of scarring of the
    liver, 23–24
HLA locus on chromosome 6, 9, 17
Homozygote, 35
Hormonal production, 74
Human Genome Project, 30
Hydration, 81
Hydrochlorothiazide, 97
Hyperferritinemia, 12

I

Iceland, occurrence in, 2, 4
Impotence, 6, 68, 74
Imuran, 183
Infection, susceptibility to, 77, 185
Initial screening procedures, 18
Iron
    absorption, 9, 80–81
    accumulation, stages of, 67

deficiency, 3
defined, 10
dietary role, 80
role of, 1–2
supplementation, 63–64
tests for, 15–17
Iron chelation therapy, 149–150
Iron depletion therapy, 148
Iron Disorders Institute, Inc., 202
Iron overload, 11, 12, 160, 200
Iron Overload Disease Association,
    Inc., 203
Iron studies, 28, 67–68
Islet cells, damage of, 73

J

Jaundice, 26, 69–70
Joint involvement, 29
Journal writing, 120
Juvenile hemochromatosis, 12

K

Klebsiella, 77

L

Laboratory tests, normal and abnormal
    values for, 25
Lasix, 97
Lethargy, 6, 68
Listeria, 77
Liver, role of the, 2, 90–93
Liver biopsy, 20–21, 147
Liver blood tests, 24–28
Liver cancer
    advanced stage, 166

alcohol injection, 169
chemoembolization, 168
chemotherapy, 169
considerations, 156–157
cryosurgery, 169
early stage, 165
hepatic resection, 166
high-frequency radio waves, treat-
    ment with, 168
metastatic liver cancer, 166
primary liver cancer (hepatoma),
    158
radiofrequency tumor ablation, 168
risk factors, 159–161
secondary liver cancer, 158
statistical implications, 158–159
testing procedures, 163–165
transplantation, 167–168 (See also
    Transplantation)
treatment, 165–169
warning signs, 162–163
Liver disease, 7, 69–72, 159–160
Liver enzymes, 24–26
Liver imaging tests, 18
Liver scarring, stages of, 23–24
Liver shunt, 70
Living-donor liver transplant, 179–181

M

Magnesium deficiency, 96
Magnetic resonance imaging (MRI),
    18, 19–20, 164
Maintenance therapy, 148–149
Managed care options, 128–129
Medicaid, 132
Medicare, 132
Meditation, use of, 120
Melanesian iron overload, 12
MELD score. See Model for End-stage
    Liver Disease score
Memory lapse, 6

Mental alterations, 69, 71–72

Metabolic function, impairment of, 72

Metastatic liver cancer, 166

Metolozone, 97

Midamor, 97

Model for End-stage Liver Disease score, 191

Mucor species, 77

Muscle ache, 6, 68

Mutations. *See also* specific mutations
  carriers, 11
  C282Y, 4, 9, 17, 18, 34, 48
  H63D, 9, 17, 48
  one mutated gene, 10
  S65C, 48
  two mutated genes (HH), 10

Mycophenolate mofetil, 183, 186

N

National Association for Rare Disorders, Inc., 204

National Institutes of Health (NIH), 204–205

National Society of Genetic Counselors, Inc., 204

Needle aspiration of joint fluid, 29

Neonatal hemochromatosis, 12

Neoral, 183

Non-alcoholic fatty liver. *See* Fatty liver

Non-cirrhotic patients
  caloric requirements, 93–94
  vitamin supplementation, 94

Normal values for laboratory testing, 25

North European descent, frequency in, 2, 4, 50

Nutritional considerations
  absorption of iron, 80–81
  alcohol usage, 83
  apple juice, drinking of, 82

  balanced diet, eating a, 81, 88–90
  bile, role of, 92
  body weight, ideal, 87–88
  carbohydrate metabolism, 91
  cast-iron skillets, use of, 83
  cirrhotic patients, 94–97
  fat metabolism, 92
  fluids, drinking of, 81
  food labels, importance of, 82
  fruits and vegetables, eat, 82
  hepatitis vaccinations, 82
  iron, role of dietary, 80
  liver, role of the, 90–93
  non-cirrhotic patients, 93–94
  patient suggestions, 84–87
  protein metabolism, 91–92
  raw shellfish, 84
  red meat, reduction of, 82
  smoking, 83
  tea, drinking of, 82
  Vitamin B complex, 82
  vitamin supplementation, 83, 93
  water content, review of, 82
  weight loss, 83

O

Occurrence of, 2–3, 4–5

One gene, mutation of, 4

One mutated gene, 10

Ongoing medical care costs, 125–127

Organ allocation, 191–192

Organ damage, 2

Organ dysfunction, 6, 68

Organ function, 32

Origination of, 2–3

Osteopenia, 76

Osteoporosis, 76

P

Pancreatic dysfunction, 73
Percutaneous biopsy procedure, 21–23
Phenotype, relationship between geno-
    type and, 195
Phlebotomy, 2, 124–125, 144–147
Portal hypertension, 27
Prednisone, 183, 186
Premenopausal first-degree relatives, 18
Primary liver cancer (hepatoma), 158
Private health insurance, 127–131
Prograf, 183
Progression of hemochromatosis, 7
Protein metabolism, 91–92
Proteins, role of, 34
Prothrombin time, 27
PT. *See* Prothrombin time

R

Radiofrequency tumor ablation, 168
Radiologic findings, 29, 164
Rapamune, 183, 186
Raw shellfish, 84
Reddening of the palms, 69
Red meat, reduction of, 82
Rejection, prevention of, 183–185, 185
Relaxation techniques, use of, 120
Research trends
    animal and cell culture models,
        200–201
    cost-effectivness of screening,
        197–198
    DMT1, 200
    ferrireductase (Dcytb), 200
    ferroportin 1 (FP1), 200
    genotype and phenotype, relation-
        ship between, 195
    hepcidin, 200
    HFE research, 200

    iron overload, stages to, 200
    screening implications, 198
    screening procedures, optimal,
        195–196
    study subject, volunteering as a,
        198–199
    transferrin and transferrin receptor,
        200
Rhizopus, 77
RNA, role of, 34

S

Salmonella, 77
Salt restriction, 70
Sandimmune, 183
S65C, 48
Screening implications and procedures,
    195–196, 198
Screening procedures, 18
Secondary liver cancer, 158
Serum iron, 16
Serum transferrin saturation, 28
Sexual dysfunction, 6, 74
Sheldon, Joseph H., 8
Short-term disability leave, 133—134
Sirolimus, 183, 186
Skin pigmentation, 8, 9, 68, 75
Smoking, 83
Social security disability insurance,
    135–136
Solumedrol, 183
Spider telangiectasia, 69
Spiritual self, finding your, 120–121
Spironolactone, 97
Stages of liver scarring, histologic,
    23–24
Starzl, Dr. Thomas, 172, 181
Steatohepatitis, 69
Stercobilin, 26
Steroids, 183
Study subject, volunteering as a,

198–199
Supplemental security income, 136–137
Support groups, use of, 116–118, 177–178
Swelling of the ankles or abdomen, 6
Symptoms
  abdominal discomfort, 6, 68
  abnormal liver tests, 68, 69
  apathy, 6, 68
  arthritis, 6, 76
  ascites, 70, 173
  bone thinning, 76
  bronze tone to skin, 6, 68, 75
  bruising, 6, 69
  cardiac dysfunction, 72–73
  cirrhosis (See Cirrhosis)
  concentration, lack of, 6
  confusion, periods of, 6
  diabetes mellitus, 6, 68, 73, 75
  dilated capillaries, 69
  edema, 70
  encephalopathy, 71–72, 173
  endocrine system dysfunction, 73–75
  energy, lack of, 5, 6, 68
  fatigue, 5, 6, 68
  fluid accumulation, 69
  fluid in the lungs or other organs, 6
  heart, complications of the, 6, 68, 72–73
  impotence, 6, 68, 74
  infection, susceptibility to, 77
  islet cells, damage of, 73
  jaundice, 69–70
  lethargy, 6, 68
  memory lapse, 6
  mental alterations, 69, 71–72
  metabolic function, impairment of, 72
  muscle ache, 6, 68
  organ dysfunction, 6, 68
  osteopenia, 76
  osteoporosis, 76

  pancreatic dysfunction, 73
  reddening of the palms, 69
  sexual dysfunction, 6, 74
  skin pigmentation, 68, 75
  spider telangiectasia, 69
  swelling of the ankles or abdomen, 6
  synthetic function, impairment of, 72
  varices, 70–71, 173
  weakness, 6, 68
  weight loss, 6, 68
  yellowing of the whites of eyes, 6, 69
Synthetic function, impairment of, 72

T

Tacrolimus, 183, 186
Tea, drinking of, 82
Testing for hemochromatosis
  albumin, 26–27
  alpha-fetoprotein, 27, 164
  bilirubin, 26
  cardiac catheterization, 28
  cardiac studies, 28
  clotting factors, 27
  complete blood count (CBC), 27–28
  computed tomography (CT), 18, 19, 165
  echocardiogram, 28
  endocrine testing, 29
  endomyocardial biopsy, 28
  ferritin, 16–17, 18
  gene testing, 17–18
  HLA testing, 17
  initial screening procedures, 18
  iron, tests for, 15–17, 28
  joint involvement, 29
  liver biopsy, 20–21
  liver blood tests, 24–28
  liver enzymes, 24–26

liver imaging tests, 18
magnetic resonance imaging (MRI),
    18, 19–20, 164
needle aspiration of joint fluid, 29
percutaneous biopsy procedure,
    21–23
radiologic findings, 29, 164
serum iron, 16
serum transferrin saturation, 28
total iron binding capacity (TIBC),
    16
transferrin saturation, 16, 18
transjugular biopsy procedure, 23
ultrasonography, 18–19, 164
Theological challenges, 121
Thomas, W., 9
TIBC. See Total iron binding capacity
TIPS. See Transjugular intrahepatic
    portal-systemic shunt
Total iron binding capacity, 16
Transferrin, 15
Transferrin and transferrin receptor,
    200
Transferrin saturation, 16, 18, 147
Transjugular biopsy procedure, 23
Transjugular intrahepatic portal-sys-
    temic shunt, 70
Transmission of mutations in families,
    35
Transplantation
    candidacy, 173
    carriers, issues relevant to C282Y,
        190–191
    centers for excellence, 192
    complications, management of, 185
    denial of, 174
    development of, 172–173
    donor livers, 178–179
    evaluation process, 175–176
    hospital stay, post-operative,
        182–183
    indicators of, 173–174
    infection, 185
    living-donor liver transplant,
        179–181
    organ allocation, 191–192
    psychological considerations,
        186–188
    rejection, prevention of, 183–185,
        185
    side effects of medications, 185–186
    support groups, 177–178
    surgical procedure, 181–182
    survival rates, 188–190
    team, transplant, 175
    waiting list, 176–177
Transplant Recipients International
        Organization, Inc., 205
Treatment
    challenges to treatment, 150–151
    costs (See Financial considerations)
    iron chelation therapy, 149–150
    iron depletion therapy, 148
    maintenance therapy, 148–149
    patient suggestions, 151–153
    phlebotomy, 144–147
Trousseau, Armand, 8
Tsuchihashi, Z., 9
Two mutated genes (HH), 4, 10

U

Ultrasonography, 18–19, 164
United Network for Organ-Sharing,
        191, 205
UNOS. See United Network for
        Organ-Sharing
Urine, darkening of the, 26

V

Varices, 70–71, 173
Veterans Administration, 132
Vibrio vulnificus, 77

Viral hepatitis, 7, 12
Visualization, use of, 120
Vitamin B complex, 82
Vitamin C supplementation, 63–64, 83
Vitamin K, administration of, 27
Vitamin supplementation, 83, 93
Von Recklinghausen, H., 8, 9

W

Waiting list, 176–177
Water content, review of, 82
Weakness, 6, 68
Weight loss, 6, 68, 83
Women, implications for, 6, 8

Y

Yellowing of the whites of eyes, 6, 26, 69
Yersinia enterocolitica, 77

Z

Zaroxylyn, 97
Zinc deficiency, 96

Healthy Living Books

Healthy Living Books brings together recognized experts from the fields of health, medicine, fitness, and nutrition to provide millions of men and women with the reliable information they need to lead longer, healthier lives.

Our editors recognize that good health comes from healthy lifestyle choices: eating well, exercising regularly, and preventing illness through sound knowledge and intelligent action.

In this day and age, when fewer people are covered by health insurance and more face increased health risks due to sedentary lifestyles, improper nutrition, and the challenges of aging, there is a profound need for solid, tested guidance. That's where we fit in.

Our medical team consists of physicians and specialists from the country's leading medical centers and institutions. Our recipes are kitchen-tested for reliability and include nutritional analysis so that home cooks will find it easy to put delicious, healthful meals on the table. Our exercise programs are prepared by nationally certified personal trainers and rehabilitation experts. All titles are presented in clear, concise language that makes reading fun and useful.

Visit our Website at www.healthylivingbooks.com

Healthy Living Books has something for everyone.